D1236778

THE AMERICAN

FLUORIDATION

EXPERIMENT

THE AMERICAN

FLUORIDATION

EXPERIMENT

By F. B. EXNER, M.D.

and

G. L. WALDBOTT, M.D.

Edited by

JAMES RORTY

THE DEVIN-ADAIR COMPANY, NEW YORK
1957

First Printing: March 1957
Second Printing: June 1957

Canadian Agents: Thomas Nelson & Sons, Ltd., Toronto

Library of Congress Catalogue Card No.: 56-12140
Printed in the United States of America

CONTENTS

THE AMERICAN

FLUORIDATION

EXPERIMENT

INTRODUCTION

TWENTY-EIGHT MILLION

HUMAN GUINEA PIGS

BY JAMES RORTY

AT this writing, some twenty-eight million Americans have been using artificially fluoridated public water supplies for varying periods, ranging from eleven years to a few months. They are willing or unwilling guinea pigs in what many American scientists and most Europeans regard as a huge, unprecedented, and possibly disastrous national experiment.

Hitherto, public health administration, involving as it does the health and welfare of millions of people, has not been regarded as a proper field for medical experimentation. This is the first time that the United States Public Health Service has ventured to use public water systems as a vehicle for the random treatment of whole populations with a dangerous drug, known to be cumulatively poisonous even when consumed in minute quantities.

1

In at least four respects the fluoridation program for the prevention of tooth decay in young children must be considered experimental and without precedent:

1. It represents an unprecedented enlargement of the responsibility and authority of the Public Health Service.

2. It subjects the entire urban population to treatment with a medication designed to benefit only a comparative few.

3. The program provides no adequate control of the dosage with respect to the requirements and tolerances of individual patients, who may be young or old, well or sick, allergic or malnourished.

4. The results of the treatment cannot be predicted, since by its own admission the Public Health Service has conducted no adequate preliminary studies of the effects of artificially fluoridated water on children and none whatever of the effects upon adults. Authorities agree that, although other organs are affected sooner, it takes from ten to twenty-five years for the cumulative effects of fluorides on bones to manifest themselves. Hence, not until 1965, at least, will it be known whether fluoridation is either safe or genuinely efficacious.

There is perhaps a fifth respect in which the program is unique and experimental. This is the first time that the official sponsors of a public-health measure have censored, intimidated, and regimented the interested health professions. It is the first time that public-health officials have deliberately falsified, distorted, and suppressed scientific evidence tending to impugn the safety of a public-health measure. It is the first time that the sponsors of such a program have systematically slandered its professional and lay critics and opponents.

Fluorine Has a History

Fluorine has a history and an extensive chemical and medical literature, much of which has been ignored or suppressed by the official sponsors of the fluoridation program.

To the chemist, fluorine is the most reactive of the elements, combining violently with whatever it contacts, and as different from its milder cousins, chlorine, bromine, and iodine, as a tiger from tabby cats. Its acids (hydrofluoric and hydrofluosilicic) are only slightly less destructive, creating havoc with equipment, and lethal in smallest quantity. Their salts, the fluorides, are still among the most toxic of substances, efficient poisons for rats or roaches—or for humans.

To the veterinarian and the physician, fluorine is known chiefly through the classic work of K. Roholm, the Danish investigator. Twenty years ago Roholm described the effects on animals and human beings of fluorine fumes discharged by aluminum, steel, and fertilizer plants, and revealed the hazards to workers exposed to fluorine poisoning in industry.

Neither Roholm nor the public-health authorities then contemplated using fluorides for the indiscriminate medication of urban populations. The problem, as they saw it, was to get fluorine out of the animal and human environment, not to put it in. Indeed, that was the problem as it was seen by the American discoverers of the relationship between the presence of natural fluorides in drinking water and the phenomenon, familiar for many decades to the early settlers of our Southwest, known as "mottled teeth" or "Texas teeth."

Today the elimination of fluorine from the public water supply, or the procurement of fluorine-free water from independent sources, remains the problem in many areas of the Southwest, where mottled teeth are common. Artificial dentures are also common in these areas, because fluorine increases the incidence of periodontal disease (gingivitis and pyorrhea) and when the brittle, fluorized teeth decay, as they do, it is often impossible to repair them.

FLUORINE OR CALCIUM?

The discovery that "mottled teeth" were fluorized teeth is credited to Margaret C. and H. V. Smith, biochemists at the University of Arizona. The mottling appears first as dull white flecks on the surface of the translucent enamel, making the teeth look unnatural. The effect is seen only in people who have lived in fluorine areas throughout their childhood, but since the mottling of the growing teeth in childhood becomes darker with age, it often results in permanent disfigurement.

Studies conducted during the twenties under the sponsorship of the American Dental Association showed a relationship between the hardness of fluorine-containing water and the incidence of mottling; the more calcium the less mottling. During the thirties the epidemiological surveys of the Public Health Service tended to confirm this finding; studies which appeared to show an inverse relationship between the incidence of tooth decay in young children and the amount of fluorine in the water revealed an even closer correlation between tooth decay and the amount of calcium and other minerals in the water; the more calcium the fewer cavities.

In their initial attempts to apply the caries-fluorine relationship, dentists painted the teeth of young children with fluoride salts and obtained, according to some reports, an average reduction of 40 percent in the incidence of tooth decay, and according to others, little or no improvement. The difficulty and expensiveness of the treatment limited its usefulness; in New York the Guggenheim Dental Clinic abandoned the topical application of fluoride when it was found that an equal expenditure for repair work resulted in more net improvement of the children's teeth.

ORIGIN OF THE FLUORIDATION THESIS

The first suggestion that fluorine might be added to water supplies as a means of obtaining a general reduction of tooth decay among young children appeared in 1939, in a paper by Dr. G. J. Cox, then a research fellow at the Mellon Institute in Pittsburgh. In this paper, Dr. Cox suggested that "in addition to adding fluoride to water, other media such as bottled water, milk supply and fluorine-containing medicinals are feasible."

A few years later the general public got an anticipatory intimation of the water-fluoridation idea when Hereford, in Deaf Smith County, Texas, was publicized in an article in *Collier's* magazine, reprinted in the February 1943 issue of *The Reader's Digest* as "The Town without a Toothache." Hereford's water supply contained from 1.5 to 2.5 parts per million of fluorine, as well as unusually high amounts of calcium and other mineral solids.

Dr. C. W. Heard, the local dentist whose "no business" report had started the publicity, accepted with some reservations the idea that the fluorine content of the water was the sole or even the chief cause of the relatively low incidence of tooth decay in Hereford and Deaf Smith County. He suspected, with reason, that the comparatively good dental health of his townsfolk was more properly attributable to a number of other factors, such as the high mineralization of both the water and the soil of Deaf Smith County and the high mineral content of the food products grown on that soil. The locally produced wheat, milk, meat, and vegetables were analyzed and all were found to be exceptionally high in phosphorus, as well as calcium, iron, magnesium, and trace minerals.

The pioneers who ate these highly mineralized foods tended to have good teeth, but with the coming of progress and a change to a more sophisticated diet of white flour, sugar, and other processed foods, the picture changed. In 1951 Dr. Heard wrote, in a pamphlet issued by the Lee Foundation for Nutritional Research:

> It is not true that Hereford, Texas, is a town without a toothache. This phrase has been used effectively by people interested in marketing sodium fluoride all over the country.
>
> I have practiced dentistry here for years and incidence of tooth decay originally was very low. Considerable research

by some dental authorities brought the suggestion that the relatively high content of natural fluorine in the water might be the reason. I accepted this conclusion for a time.

However, as the town grew and people began to live on processed foods . . . tooth decay increased by leaps and bounds. The increase persisted in spite of the fact that the people were drinking the same water they drank when they were eating natural and unadulterated foods.

The dental investigators made a serious mistake when they gave fluorine the credit for our good teeth. They overlooked the food grown in our rich, well-mineralized soil. It is these minerals, of which processed food robs the body, that build health and good teeth. That goes for trace minerals as well as for nitrogen, calcium, potash, and phosphorus. It takes all these elements to build sound bodies. . . ."

Too Much Sugar Causes Tooth Decay

Dr. Heard's belief that the chief cause of tooth decay is dietary is shared by most medical and dental authorities. Prior to the launching of the fluoridation campaign, this was the accepted view of both the Public Health Service and of the American Dental Association, later to become the most ardent proponent of the fluoridation thesis. The cause-and-effect relationship between the excessive consumption of vitamin- and mineral-deficient foods and the increasing ravages of tooth decay in all the industrialized and urbanized countries of the world is shown by a mass of evidence compiled by research dentists, nutritionists, physicians, and epidemiologists. Of the many lessons taught our public health workers by World War II, none was more striking than the evidence, pouring in from embattled Europe, that the wartime rationing of sugar had contributed importantly to a coincident drop in the incidence of tooth decay among children.

The war had barely ended when Schour and Massler reported that the relatively sugarless population of wartime Italy had from one half to one seventh as much tooth decay as the average for sugar-saturated America, which had reduced sugar consumption rather little during the war. In hard-pinched Norway, tooth decay among school children dropped by half. Norwegian dentists agreed that this was due to the wartime shortage of refined carbohydrates, especially sugar.

In America the official press of the American Dental Association printed these findings. The same thing had happened during World War I, and the cause-and-effect relationship had been confirmed by many controlled studies, some of them sponsored by the ADA itself. Indeed, American dentists scarcely needed the studies to convince them that the indulged "sweet tooth" of the American child was a major cause of the increasing prevalence of tooth decay in the American population. Practicing dentists, like the celebrated Dr. Fred Miller, of Altoona, Pennsylvania, crusaded actively against the tooth-destroying dietary habits of the average American family. Again and again they proved that children brought up on good natural foods and without candy, pastries, and soft drinks often had perfect teeth on attaining adulthood.

Thus, in 1950, the reduction of sugar intake, in the diet of children especially, was second only to tooth brushing in the credo of prevention-minded American dentists. Yet it was in that year that the American Dental Association suddenly turned its face away from the admitted prime cause of tooth decay and chose instead to promote a program of mass medication of dubious effectiveness and even more dubious safety. The program, which was sanctioned by the United States Public Health Service after only five years of a scheduled ten-year tryout in the pilot-plant cities of Grand Rapids, Michigan, and Newburgh, New York, was the fluoridation of municipal water supplies.

THE FLUORIDATION BANDWAGON

In November 1950 the American Dental Association joined the parade of professional societies endorsing the program.* It

* The February 1951 edition of a Public Health Service booklet entitled "Better Health for 5 to 14 Cents a Year through Fluoridated Water" lists the early endorsements as follows:

was quickly followed by the American Public Health Association, the National Research Council, and the American Medical Association (which, however, limited its approval to an endorsement of the "principle" of fluoridation). Among the earliest advocates of the program was the Sugar Research Foundation, which is the research and propaganda arm of the sugar-refining industry. The Foundation had been giving generous support to *ad hoc* investigations to show that America's 100-pound-per-capita annual consumption of sugar was not excessive. (Most nutritionists who have not been embarrassed by the Sugar Research Foundation's grants agree that this is at least three times too much.) In the October 1949 issue of the Foundation's publication, *The Sugar Molecule,* its scientific director, Dr. Robert C. Hockett, acknowledged unblushingly that the purpose of the dental-caries research was "to find out how tooth decay may be controlled effectively without restriction of sugar intake."

The fluoridation program was admirably designed to ward off nutritional criticism of sugar. It gave dentists something to talk about other than what every dentist knew, namely that less sugar in a child's diet meant less decay. State and local dental societies were mobilized in support of fluoridation, and dissenters were silenced by an unprecedented gag rule that penalized by expulsion any public criticism of fluoridation. The official dental press was closed to critics of the program. Similar

1 American Water Works Association, June 1, 1949.
2 State and Territorial Dental Health Directors, June 8, 1950.
3 Public Health Service, June 22, 1950.
4 American Association of Public Health Dentists, October 29, 1950.
5 American Dental Association, October 30–November 2, 1950.
6 State and Territorial Health Officers, November 1950.
7 American Public Health Association, November 1950.

Since later editions of this booklet list the PHS endorsement as 1951, it would seem that after giving the program an initial push through its own action and that of the State and Territorial Dental Health Directors, the Public Health Service climbed down off its own bandwagon and then climbed aboard again a year later. The early action of the American Waterworks Association was not a genuine endorsement (see chapter 7) but merely a permissive resolution slipped through at a national convention, despite the fact that the majority of water engineers then, as now, opposed the program.

and only slightly less effective pressure was exerted upon the medical profession and its official press.

THE "ENGINEERING OF CONSENT"

A high-pressure propaganda bureau, with offices in the Chicago headquarters of the American Dental Association, generated a flood of "educational" literature, of planted articles, of broadcasts teeming with half truths, outright falsifications, and slander of lay and professional opponents. Opposition to fluoridation, declared its official advocates, was confined to "food faddists, purveyors of so-called health foods, publicity seekers, and writers of 'sensation' articles, together with a very few members of the health professions."

That opposition is substantial, has been steadily increasing, and is effective whenever it can make itself heard. At the 1951 hearings of the Delaney Committee to Investigate the Use of Chemicals in Food and Cosmetics, six distinguished scientists were summoned by the Committee, namely, Robert S. Harris, Ph.D., Director of the Nutritional Biochemistry Laboratories of the Massachusetts Institute of Technology; E. B. Hart, Sc.D., professor of biochemistry, University of Wisconsin, Hans H. Neumann, M.D., research assistant in dental research, Columbia University; Howard V. Smith, associate agricultural chemist, University of Arizona; Margaret C. Smith, Ph.D., formerly head of the department of human nutrition, University of Arizona, and Alfred Taylor, Ph.D., Biochemical Institute, University of Texas.

CONGRESS WARNS: "GO SLOW"

They testified so convincingly against the program that the Committee, in its final report, declared unanimously that "a sufficient number of unanswered questions concerning the safety of the (fluoridation) program exists to warrant a conservative attitude." In a supplementary statement, Congressman A. L. Miller, a medical doctor and former health director of the state of Nebraska, asserted:

"I am convinced that many of the groups who now endorse fluorides in water are merely parroting each other's opinions. They have done no original research themselves."

Normally, an adverse Congressional report such as this might have been expected to lead to the suspension and reexamination of the program. Instead, the public-health and dental fluoridators redoubled their promotional efforts.

As long ago as May 1955, according to the Public Health Service, the water supplies of 1085 communities, with a population of nearly 21 million, were being fluoridated. But to balance this, 40 million Americans in over 500 cities had either rejected the program or, having tried it, had abandoned it and junked their fluoridation equipment. Among the cities and towns (approximately 75 at this writing) that have abandoned the program after brief trials are San Diego, California; Akron, Ohio; Saginaw, Michigan; Northampton and Williamstown, Massachusetts; Baton Rouge, Louisiana; Grosse Pointe, Michigan.

The City Council of Newark, N. J., voted to adopt the alternative "pill" program proposed by B. C. Nesin, director of the laboratories of New York City's Department of Water, Gas and Electricity (See Chapter 8). This program permits a controlled dosage of fluoride, at the option of the parents. It involves relatively little hazard to the children and none to adults, and costs a fraction of what is required to install and service fluoridation of the water supply. Incidentally, the suppliers of fluorides, who, along with the manufacturers of fluoridation equipment, are among the most active promoters of the program, have more than doubled their prices since the initiation of the pilot-plant demonstrations in 1945. Among these suppliers are Dupont, the Aluminum Company of America, and General Chemical Company, New York.

Europe Watches "the American Experiment"

Despite the promotional efforts of representatives of the Public Health Service who have traveled and lectured in behalf of fluoridation, the program has made little headway abroad. In January 1955 the dentists of France at their annual convention voted against the program after the Institut Pasteur and the Ministry of Health had failed to approve it. Switzerland is going slow on the program as a result of experiments which indicate that fluorine may aggravate thyroid imbalance in persons suffering from goiter. Concerning the status of the fluoridation program in Switzerland, Dr. T. Gordonoff, of Berne, writes:

> In several parts of our country, children receive tablets with fluorine, but the fluoridation of drinking water has not been accomplished. We trust it will not happen in view of the special circumstances here regarding our thyroid problem.
>
> Twenty years ago our population had many goiters— they have disappeared because of iodized salt. Research here demonstrates clearly an antagonism between iodine and fluorine. . . . We also showed in another experiment that the calcium metabolism is greatly affected by fluorine. Since the bone picks up 30 percent less calcium in the presence of fluorine, the danger of osteoporosis (softening of the bone) in a growing organism is very very great.* (*National Fluoridation News,* April 1955.)

In Sweden, the Scientific Council has prohibited all fluoridation of water supplies pending further study. This decision followed an adverse report by the Royal Medical Board issued on February 25, 1955, and reported in the March 2, 1955, issue of the Stockholm *Dagens Nyheter.* The Board stated that as long as full knowledge as to the desirable medical effects is not at hand, it prefers to wait for complete reports of "the American experiment."

In England, where a few fluoridation experiments were begun, following the visit to this country of a British mission of inquiry, the fluoridation program has run into increasing opposition from both health professionals and laymen. In the February 12, 1955, issue of the *British Medical Journal,* Dr. Hugh Sinclair, director

---

* The precise effect of fluorine on goiter remains to be determined.

of Oxford University's Laboratory of Human Nutrition, declared that "the Health Ministry's plan to put chemicals called fluorides into drinking water may poison millions of people." Dr. Sinclair believes that fluorides may be more dangerous in Britain than in the United States, because most Britains eat more fish and drink more tea than do Americans—and both fish and tea are rich in fluorine; also because of the considerable content of fluorine in the polluted air of British industrial centers.

On December 3, 1955, the *London Times* gave editorial expression to the prevailing British attitude toward "the American experiment." Said the *Times:*

> . . . Before decisions are taken, and especially if there are to be experiments, it would seem desirable that there should be more open consultation and more discussion than there has been. An argument brought forward that since fluorides are found in most water and the practice proposed is merely to bring the poor-quality water up to the standard of the best, and that this differentiates the proposal from others to introduce wholly new elements into water for the purpose of mass prophylaxis, has no real validity. The issue of principle is the same whether "additives" are already in the water in small quantities or not. Experts are too readily persuaded both that what they propose is of great importance and that the public is too stupid to realize it. It is an attitude likely to recoil on those who adopt it.

What the *Times* predicted has in fact happened. In several of the British pilot-plant communities, the protests of the townspeople, led by the British Housewives League, have forced suspension of the experiments.

Adverse Findings Accumulate

The most alarming aspect of the fluoridation program is the reckless arrogance, obstinacy, and unscrupulousness of the United

States Public Health Service in continuing to promote the program while ignoring and, where possible, suppressing evidence that it is neither safe nor genuinely efficacious. Even in 1950, when our Washington bureaucracy gave the program the green light, much of this evidence was already in the scientific literature. Since then, while foreign health authorities have been marking time, waiting for the results of "the American experiment," new evidence has poured in, all of it tending to show that fluoridation was indeed an experiment and that the findings to date are unfavorable.

Evidence comes from physicians in the fluoridated cities and from their patients, who became ill drinking fluoridated water; the patients exhibited the classic symptoms of fluorine poisoning, and recovered when they stopped.

Evidence comes from practicing dentists in the fluoridated cities who failed to find in the fluorized teeth of their young patients the reduction in caries they had been told to expect. What they *are* finding is that the mottling effect of fluoridation in the test cities, some of it so severe as to be disfiguring, is running as high as thirty percent instead of the predicted ten-percent "unobjectionable" mottling.

Evidence comes from food processors and pharmaceutical firms caught between the Food and Drug Administration, which sets "tolerance limits" for the amount of fluorine their products may contain, and the Public Health Service, which, by fluoridating the public water supplies on which they are dependent, forces them to use deep wells or to defluorinate at great expense the water used in their processing operations.

Evidence comes from breeders of dogs and chinchillas which have failed to reproduce and have died in numbers as a result of their involuntary subjection to the fluoridation experiment.

Evidence comes from water engineers all over the country who report corroded and clogged fluoridating equipment; who say that it is impossible to control accurately the amount of fluorine introduced into the water supply or to prevent the "fall out" and accumulation of dangerous fluoride deposits in the system.

It comes, finally, from specialized scientists here and abroad;

allergists, endocrinologists, toxicologists, biochemists, bio-statisticians, research dentists. Knowing something about the ramified and insidious effects of fluorine as a cumulative systemic poison, these independent investigators refused to accept as final the statement of the American Dental Association that "twenty years of scientific data have established beyond a reasonable doubt the safety and effectiveness of fluoridation."

In the library, these scientists checked the official assurance that there is nothing in the literature to indicate any danger from fluorine in the water supply at one part per million, and that the factor of safety provided for by the program is ample. They found to their amazement that the literature is full of reports showing serious damage both to teeth and to the general health from fluorine at or near the recommended level, and that the factor of safety is nonexistent.

They found not only that the DMF (decayed, missing, filled) rate employed by the official dental examiners is a notoriously unreliable yardstick for the measurement of dental decay (no two dental examiners have ever been known to come up with the same finding) but that, to obtain a paper reduction of 60 percent in the incidence of tooth decay, the Public Health Service has stretched this rubber yardstick in a manner calculated to astonish and appall any reputable bio-statistician. (See Appendix 3, page 244.)

They found that the Public Health Service has scrapped the pilot-plant findings (in Ottawa, Kansas, and Evanston, Illinois) when they haven't fitted the fluoridation thesis; that it has suppressed the results of some government surveys and falsified the results of others.

The Spread of Fluorine Poisoning

In all the fluoridated cities, health officials have insisted on regarding the fluoridation thesis as proved and its critics as crackpots. Otherwise they might have learned much by observing the effects of fluoridation on the populations involved, as related to the wide and often critical differences in the total mineral content of the fluoridated water, and to the cases of fluoride intoxication reported by Drs. Waldbott, Wolf, Feltman, and other highly qualified and responsible investigators.

Fluorine poisoning approaching epidemic proportions was first reported from Saginaw, Michigan, which adopted fluoridation in 1950 and discontinued the program in 1954. Saginaw's water supply is exceptionally soft, containing only 16.8 parts per million of calcium.

As early as 1925, Dr. C. A. Pierle, in a study sponsored by the American Dental Association, established the relationship between mottled teeth and calcium deficiency. Dr. Pierle noted that mottling was prevalent in areas where the drinking water contained little calcium, but that even in these areas, students who ate a calcium-rich diet of eggs, green vegetables, and milk three times a day rarely had mottled teeth. At that time the role of fluorine in mottling was unknown. Many other reports have noted a relationship among the incidence of fluorosis, the calcium and other mineral content of the water, and the amount of calcium in the diet.

Cases of fluorine poisoning have been reported from many of the fluoridated cities, including Coeur d'Alene, Idaho; Evanston, Illinois; San Francisco, California; Saginaw and Highland Park, Michigan; Wichita Falls, Texas, and many others. But since the Public Health Service denies the possibility of any adverse effects from fluoridation at the one-part-per-million level and refuses to concede that the program is still experimental, although it has conducted no adequate controlled studies of children or adults even in the pilot-plant cities of Grand Rapids, Michigan, and Newburgh, New York, local and state health officials have refused to take these reports seriously. (See Chapters 5 and 6.)

In 1952, Congressman Miller of Nebraska, a member of the Delaney Committee, called attention to a possible relationship between the official start of fluoridation in Grand Rapids in 1945 (or in 1941, if former Mayor George W. Welsh is to be believed) and a sudden rise in the mortality from cardio-vascular diseases, cancer, intracranial lesions, and diabetes.

Dr. W. B. Prothro, the county-city health officer, at first denied that there had been any significant rise in the mortality of the Grand Rapids population from the major degenerative diseases. Not until July 1955 was it officially acknowledged that Congressman Miller had been right all the time: that in 1950 the Grand Rapids mortality from these diseases ran from 20 to 40 percent above the state averages. While continuing to insist that these figures could bear no possible relation to fluoridation, Dr. Prothro announced that his department would spend $5,000 in an attempt to find the explanation.

In 1953 Newburgh health statistics, too, showed an abnormal and suspicious rise in the mortality from heart disease. According to the first nationwide report since 1949, Newburgh had 882 deaths from heart disease per 100,000, compared to an average for the Middle Atlantic States of 590 and a national average of 507. Again the Public Health Service denied any possible connection between these figures and the fluoridation of Newburgh's water supply in 1945.

IS DENTAL CARIES REALLY BEING REDUCED IN THE FLUORIDATED CITIES?

Apart from the moot question of safety, there is good reason to doubt that the fluoridation experiment to date has produced *any* net improvement of the dental—and periodontal—health of children or adults.

Critics of the program have expressed the following reasons for challenging the official claims of the Public Health Service and the American Dental Association:

1. There is no scientific support for the official thesis that fluorine is a "missing ingredient" which fluoridation of the water supply provides. McCollum, Maynard, Phillips, McCay, and other leading nutritionists have found no evidence to warrant the belief that fluorine in *any* quantity is essential to the human or animal organism or to the production of good teeth. Indeed, there is much evidence to refute this contention, on which the official program of "adjusting" the fluorine intake from water to one part per million is based. An unpublished Public Health

Service survey of the dental condition of the natives of American Samoa revealed a remarkably *low* incidence of tooth decay in a population whose drinking water contained practically no fluorine. On the other hand, tooth decay is frequently found to be rampant in areas where nature has "adjusted" the fluorine content of the water to what the Public Health Service considers the right level. Again and again, during the present fluoridation campaign, zealous local health officers and dentists have been made to look ridiculous when, after they had demonstrated the deplorably high prevalence of tooth decay in the child and adult population, somebody discovered belatedly that the town's water supply had always contained one part per million of fluorine or thereabouts.

Professor Alfred Kantorowicz has reported that in eighteen West German communities he could find no correlation between caries frequency and the amount of natural fluorine in the water, whereas there was a measurable improvement of the dental health of children who had been given riboflavin supplements. In the town of Hamm in Westphalia, whose water supply contains very little fluorine, the incidence of tooth decay is one fourth that of the fluoridated city of Grand Rapids. The children of Tel Aviv, whose water contains no fluorine, have far less tooth decay than the children of our fluoridated cities.

2. The findings of the public health service's examiners in the pilot-plant cities of Grand Rapids and Newburgh are subject to question on several counts. First, it is utterly unrealistic to limit the appraisal of dental health to caries. Seventy percent of tooth loss after the age of forty is caused not by caries but by periodontal disease (gingivitis, pyorrhea, etc.). Not only is there no evidence that fluorine reduces the incidence of periodontal disease, there is positive evidence that fluorine *increases* the incidence of both gingivitis and pyorrhea. In the February 1955 Journal of the Ontario (Canada) Dental Association, Dr. Keith Box pointed out that in the town of Stratford, which has been using natural-fluoride water for 37 years at 1.6 part per million, 79.2 percent of the children were found to have gingivitis, about the same as in the artificially fluoridated city of Brantford and the fluorine-free city of Sarnia. In June 1956 William F. Ram-

syer, at Cornell University, published rat studies showing a definite increase in the incidence of both gingivitis and caries in rats given fluoridated water to drink. (See Appendix 1.)

Malocclusion (crooked teeth) and gingivitis are alike ignored in the reports of the Public Health Service dental examiners in Newburgh, but both were included by the examiners of New York State's Department of Education. This undoubtedly affected the Education Department's startling findings, which were that in 1953 the proportion of Newburgh children with dental defects was 50 percent *higher* than in the fluorine-free control city of Kingston, N. Y. The school physicians of the education department employed only open-mouth tongue-blade inspection, whereas the Public Health Service dentists used mouth mirror and explorer. Hence the two examinations cannot be considered strictly comparable. However, the extreme disparity between the findings of the two sets of examiners fully warranted the question asked by Drs. Reuben Feltman, James G. Kerwin, and A. Allen London of the Hudson County, N. J., Dental Society: "Are we being confronted with a difference between cavities observed in general practice and 'statistical cavities' which required specialized interpretation of conditioned examiners?"

3. The question asked by the New Jersey critics of the fluoridation program gathers force from the fact that the DMF yardstick used by the official dental examiners is notoriously unreliable; dental examiners rarely agree on the DMF of a given child. Moreover, as Dr. Veikko Oscar Hurme, research director of the Forsythe Dental Infirmary, has pointed out, the claims for the reduction of caries in the communities now fluoridating water—from 20 to 65 percent—vary so widely as to call into question both the methods and objectivity of the examiners. Three devastating critiques of the official DMF findings in the pilot-plant cities have been published, one by Dr. M. Klerer of City College, New York, in the February-March issue of *Contemporary Issues* and another by K. K. Paluev, an engineer and statistician employed by the General Electric Company at Pittsfield, Mass., to chart the development work of the company's transformer department.

A third analysis of the Public Health Service's DMF findings in the pilot-plant cities was published by Dr. Charles Dillon in the August 1956 issue of the *Dental Digest*. Dr. Dillon points out that the only realistic measure of the improvement alleged to result from fluoridation is the increase in the percentage of sound teeth. Using the Public Health Service's own figures, he shows that the actual increase in the number of sound teeth in Newburgh was not 77.6 percent but 7.2 percent. He notes further, as does Dr. Paluev, that the percentage DMF decrease falls rapidly with advancing age, and that "in omitting to compare the rate of deterioration of the dentition before and after fluoridation, Public Health authorities have omitted to deal with perhaps the most important aspect of caries contol. . . ." All three scientists conclude that the manipulation of the data by the official Public Health Service evaluators is so flagrant as to make ridiculous the claim of an average 66-percent reduction of caries in the test cities.

In his analysis of the official findings of the Grand Rapids and Newburgh experiments (see Appendix 3), Mr. Paluev has undertaken to show that in neither city has the artificial fluoridation of the water supply prevented dental decay to any practical degree, even among eight-year-olds drinking fluoridated water from birth. What the official statistics actually show, says Mr. Paluev, is not a *reduction* but merely *a short delay in the detection* of caries. Support is lent to this conclusion by the observations of some of the dentists interviewed by the *Newburgh News* (December 14, 1955) on the occasion of the announced completion of the Newburgh experiment. None of them was prepared to confirm the official claim of a 66-percent reduction of caries. A few believed they had seen some improvement in the teeth of the younger children. One dentist testified that his youngest child, born since the start of fluoridation, had worse cavities than any of his older children. A prominent member of the Newburgh Dental Society declared that "what little effect it [fluoridation] might have had was not apparent. One effect of fluoridation, however, was abundantly manifest." Instead of the expected 10 percent "mild" and "unobjectionable" mottling, the Newburgh children born since the initiation of the program were averaging at least 30 percent mottling, some of it severe enough to become ultimately disfiguring with age.

FOOD, TOO, CONTAINS FLUORINE

Fluorine poisoning is the combined and cumulative effect of the total fluorine intake over a period of time from *all* environmental sources: water, food, and air. The effect is greater or less, hastened or delayed, depending upon the individual susceptibility of the subject. Averages mean nothing, since no two individuals drink, eat, or breathe the same amount or have average tolerances for fluorine or other poisons.

The fluorine content of foods has been studied by McClure, Monier-Williams, and others. The values found vary from a fraction of a part per million to several hundred parts, depending in some degree upon the conditions under which the foods are produced and processed. The fish foods, such as salmon, mackerel, sardines, and shrimp, are high in fluorine; the seafood diet of the Tristan da Cunha islanders probably explains the 30-percent incidence of mottled teeth of the younger people, despite the fact that the drinking water contains only 0.2 parts per million of fluorine. A meal containing fish, peas, and the usual beverage can easily account for one to three milligrams of fluorine. The fluorine content of tea may run to several hundred parts per million, and so habitual tea drinkers might be expected to exceed regularly the narrow margin of safety claimed by the proponents of the fluoridation program. The residual spray on an apple may contain one milligram of fluorine and a can of beer may contribute another milligram. Mottled teeth are common in some districts of England, where the fluorine content of the water is less than one part per million but where tea is the popular beverage. People living in fluoridated cities who eat a good deal of seafood and drink tea and beer may easily ingest a combined fluorine intake far beyond even the tolerance limits assumed by the Public Health Service.

Under the Food and Drug Law, fluorine is classified as a poison, the use of which in processed foods in any quantity is prohibited. In 1945 the Commonwealth Brewing Company was convicted and fined $5,000 for adulterating its product with fluorine.

The fluoridation of municipal water systems has multiplied the hazards against which brewers, food processors, and pharmaceutical manufacturers must safeguard their customers at any cost—and frequently the cost is heavy. In Pittsburgh, Pa., the Heinz Company is using water from its own deep wells; in Rochester, N. Y., the Beech Nut Packing Corporation is defluoridating expensively the fluoridated city water it uses in the processing of its food products.

Inevitably, food processors must concentrate the fluoridated water used in their plants, so that one part per million can become several times that in the finished product. If fluoridated water is used in yeast culturing, the fluorine content of the yeast is likely to exceed the limits considered safe by manufacturers of baby foods. If fluoridated water is used in the wet-milling of corn, the resulting concentration in corn syrup would exceed five parts per million. When the plant superintendent of a pharmaceutical manufacturer reported that the fluoridation of the city water would result in concentrating a thousandfold the fluorine content of his products, the manufacturer chose, as have many others, to shoulder the expense of defluoridating the water, declaring, "Until such time as the safety of the program is established we shall see to it that our products are free of fluorine."

THE WARNING OF THE WATER ENGINEERS

If the water engineers employed by public and private water-supply systems cannot guarantee the maintenance, with reliable accuracy, of the one-part-per-million level of fluorine dosage which the Public Health Service prescribes, then the program is not safe, regardless of all other factors.

They can give no such assurances (see Chapter 7). The majority of American water engineers have opposed the program from the beginning. Their professional publication, the *Journal of the American Water Works Association*—unlike the dental and medical press—is not censored. For years it has carried the complaints of water engineers about the difficulties and hazards of the program. Many of the towns and cities that have tried the program have been forced to abandon it by the failure of the fluoridating machinery.

Fluoridation and the Fourteenth Amendment

The right of the individual not to be subjected to medication against his will is guaranteed by the First and Fourteenth amendments of the Constitution. This right is subject only to the exercise of the state's police power to prevent "clear and present danger" to the public health. Dental caries is not a communicable disease. There can be no contention by the proponents of fluoridation that it represents a clear and present danger to the public health or that fluoridation of municipal water supplies confers its benefits, themselves questionable, upon more than a fraction of the population, namely, children under eight.

Hence, if fluoridation is defined as preventive medication or prophylaxis, which it unquestionably is, it would seem that the fluoridation program must ultimately be declared unconstitutional by the United States Supreme Court. Otherwise the Court would be obliged to reverse all previous precedents and decisions regarding the constitutional prohibition of mass medication, as qualified by the police power.

Thus far the courts of last resort have not ruled on the issue either in this country or in Canada. In a number of cases the majority opinions of the lower courts have accepted the wholly unscientific assertion of the public-health officials that fluoridation represents mere "adjustment" of the mineral content of the water supply to an "optimum" level with respect to fluorine. Hence, the lower courts have tended to sustain the right of the public-health authorities to fluoridate by the exercise of the police power, with or without a popular referendum, although even a majority popular vote for fluoridation would not invalidate the constitutional right of a minority not to be subjected to medication against its will.

That fluoridation is clearly mass medication is the view of practically all the professional health workers and water engineers who have opposed the program. On this point, Dr. V. O. Hurme, Research Director of Boston's Forsythe Dental Infirmary for Children, writes, in the June 1952 issue of *Dental Items of Interest:*

> The proponents of fluoridation have been averse to the use of the term "mass medication." Instead, they have referred to it as a "preventive procedure," a "public health measure," or the like, which is similar to chlorination of public water supplies.
>
> The dislike for the term "mass medication" is difficult to explain, inasmuch as it very accurately describes the concept underlying fluoridation. "Medicine," it is agreed, deals with the *prevention,* cure, or alleviation of disease. Prevention or alleviation of dental disease is the aim of treatment with fluorides. Vaccination, which is the medical procedure most akin to fluoridation, is for the purpose of preventing smallpox, rather than for the treatment of persons ill with the disease. It consists of introducing *into* the body a preparation which enables the body to develop immunity to a specific disease agent—the virus of smallpox.
>
> Addition of fluorides to drinking water is not for the purpose of protecting the public against any water-borne agent or agents responsible for the decay of teeth. There is no similarity here between chlorination and fluoridation. Chemically pure fluorides are drugs that are too poisonous to be dispensed to the general public over a drug store counter, at least without a prescription. Even dental hygienists have not been permitted to apply fluorides topically, without amendment of the dental laws of the states.
>
> Since "medication" refers to impregnation with anything medicinal, or with a drug or chemical, and since fluoridation is for the purpose of impregnating the public itself with

fluorides, it appears pointless to confuse the issue by deny-
ing that this novel prophylactic procedure is a form of mass
medication.

That Dr. Hurme's view is shared by at least some of the
judges who have considered the issue is indicated by the following excerpts from the dissenting opinions in the Kaul case in
Chehalis, Washington, in which the Supreme Court of the State
of Washington ruled in favor of fluoridation by a split decision
of 5 to 4.

Thus the liberty of which appellant is deprived is the right
to decide of his own free will whether he desires to apply
fluorine to his teeth for the purpose of preventing tooth decay, based upon his own opinion as to whether it would
be advantageous or disadvantageous to his personal health
—a matter, incidentally, on which there is marked and bitter
divergence of opinion within the medical and dental professions. . . . What the residents of Chehalis could not be
compelled to do one by one, it is now sought to compel
them to do *en masse*. . . . This smacks more of the police
state than of the police power. . . . The ordinance providing for fluoridation is unconstitutional on the ground that it
is an unwarranted and unjustified invasion of the liberty
guaranteed the appellant by the United States Constitution,
Amendment 14, and by our state constitution, Art. 1, Sc. 3.
[Judge Hill dissenting.]

. . . It seems to me that the principle involved is of far-
reaching consequences, because, if the city council (or
commissioners) may legally inject any such medicine into
the water, they have the right to put into it any medicinal
agent from patent medicines to antibiotics (so-called "wonder drugs") which *they* may determine from time to time
to be beneficial to the public health. . . ."
Thus will the people be deprived of a very important
part of their constitutional liberty under our republican
form of government, and the police state will be substi-

tuted for the police power of the state." [Judge Donworth dissenting.]

The alternative theory upon which the majority opinion seems to be based seeks not to disclaim compulsion, but to defend it. . . . What future proposals may be made to treat noncontagious diseases by adding ingredients to our water supply, or food, or air, only time will tell. When that day arrives, those who treasure their personal liberty will look in vain for a constitutional safeguard. The answer will be: "You gave the constitution away in the *Kaul* case." . . .

But even were it assumed that the majority of the citizens of Chehalis approve this move [fluoridation] this would not condone an impairment of constitutional rights. The constitutional guaranties are to protect the rights of the minority—not the majority. The majority does not need protection because it does not do anything it does not want to do. . . .

Can we . . . withstand the insidious erosion [of our basic liberties] produced by a multiplicity of little instances where, as here, a guaranteed right is set aside because it interferes with what is said to be good for us? [Judge Hamley dissenting.]

In Canada, two 1956 court decisions have served to slow down the campaign to fluoridate the public water supplies of Canadian cities. In the Province of New Brunswick the Supreme Court has declared that the addition of fluorine to public water supplies is illegal. In the Court's ruling, Chief Justice McNair declared that the treatment of public water supplies by chemical or other means can only be carried out as an operation for the purification of a water system or water supply. "By no stretch of the imagination," said the Court, "can that which was contemplated in respect to the Fredericton water supply, being the addition of fluoride compounds to correct a deficiency for optimum dental health, be so regarded."

In Toronto a by-law authorizing fluoridation which had been adopted by the Metropolitan Toronto Council was declared invalid by the Toronto Court of Appeal. It was expected that this decision would halt fluoridation programs in nine other communities with a total population of 200,000.

The Dilemma of the Public Health Administration

The contention of the Public Health Service and the American Dental Association that fluoridation is not experimental would be tenable only if adequate preliminary epidemiological, laboratory, and clinical studies had established the efficacy and complete safety of the program; only if the literature of fluorine poisoning contained no evidence tending to contraindicate the use of municipal water systems as vehicles for the random treatment of whole populations with fluorine; only if subsequent scientific studies had invariably confirmed the findings on which the Public Health Service based its sanction of the program; only if the application of the program in the fluoridated cities had produced no adverse effects upon the dental and general health of the populations involved, both children and adults; only if the water engineers could guarantee the accurate regulation of the fluorine dosage at one part per million.

None of these conditions can be considered fulfilled. On the contrary, the slender scientific base on which the vast inverted pyramid of fluoridation is reared has been shown to consist of inadequate, contradictory, and discredited epidemiological studies, biased and selective reviews of the literature, distorted interpretations of the Public Health Service's own findings, and a few laboratory and clinical studies which have been repeatedly discredited by subsequent investigation.

Today, a decade after the launching of the fluoridation program, it can no longer be considered even genuinely experimental. The results are in, and the findings are adverse. On the basis of Dr. Feltman's sample* (of a thousand pregnant women and

---

* Dr. Feltman's study was financed by a Public Health Service grant, which was withdrawn in 1955 when his preliminary findings not only failed

young children to whom one part per million of fluorine had been administered, eleven developed definite symptoms of fluorine poisoning), we can even estimate roughly the probable number of persons in fluoridated cities who are allergic to fluoride. It is 1.0 percent of 28,000,000, or 280,000. As for the victims of chronic fluoride poisoning who may appear ten, twenty, or thirty years from now, there is every reason to fear that their number will be far greater.

Hence, every consideration of scientific ethics, public policy, and simple humanity dictates that the experiment be discontinued and the spread of fluorine poisoning arrested before it assumes catastrophic proportions.

Shocking as the statement may sound, it is altogether probable that some, at least, of the official proponents of the program now realize this. Why, then, do they not act? Are they waiting for a face-saving alternative that will permit the gradual abandonment of water fluoridation, while diverting attention from their own criminal responsibility for endangering the health of millions? Or are they so enslaved and paralyzed by past ideological and personal commitments that they will do nothing to rescue themselves and the nation from the trap into which their arrogant folly has precipitated us?

Time will answer these questions. Meanwhile, the authors of this book can only hope for a return of sanity and courage before the most venturesome public-health experiment in history is liquidated by the undeniable realities of a national disaster.

---

to confirm the fluoridation thesis but indicated probable ill effects to a significant percentage of the population because of allergy to fluorides. (See Appendix 1.) His progress report, published in the August 1956 issue of the *Dental Digest*, described the results of administering sodium monofluorophosphate tablets, in a controlled dosage equivalent to one part per million, to pregnant women. One percent of Dr. Feltman's 1100 cases presented evidence of undesirable side effects from fluoride therapy, which subsided when the therapy was discontinued, and recurred when it was resumed. Children of the women who received fluoride showed marked delay in the eruption of the teeth, possibly because of inhibition, by the fluoride, of thyroid function. Beneficial effects in cases with hypersensitive teeth were also reported.

PART 1

FALLACIES OF THE

FLUORIDATION THESIS

BY FREDERICK B. EXNER, M.D.

FREDERICK B. EXNER, M.D.

Dr. Exner's youth was spent in Northfield, Minnesota, where his father was head of the chemistry department of Carleton College. In 1921 he was graduated from Carleton, where he majored in science and mathematics; subsequently he taught high school chemistry and physics. After postgraduate work in biology and chemistry at Carleton, he attended medical school at the University of Minnesota, graduating in 1927, and took further postgraduate work in physical chemistry and biostatistics. An internship and surgical residency was followed by two years in general practice, after which he returned to Minnesota for postgraduate work in radiology and pathology. His work on internal hernia, done at that time, is considered a classic; he also did pioneer work leading to the adoption of mass X-ray as a case-finding method for tuberculosis.

Dr. Exner has been engaged in private practice since 1933, in Seattle since 1935, as an X-ray specialist. He has served as consultant to the State Departments of Health and of Vocational Rehabilitation, and on the medical school faculty of the University of Washington. He has held numerous offices and assignments in national, state and local medical organizations.

The material in this section is the product of four years of intensive research, and is adapted from a report written for the City of New York in 1955 and published in *Northwest Medicine.*

The Physiological Action

of Fluorides

TO understand the effects of fluorides on the human body, it is first necessary to get a general idea of the processes by which such effects are produced. Full understanding would require a complete knowledge of how the body works. No one possesses such knowledge, and certainly it is not to be expected of the average reader. Nevertheless, it should be possible for everyone to understand enough so he can do his own thinking instead of trusting someone else to do it for him.

DIRECT (OR TOPICAL) VS. SYSTEMIC EFFECTS

When water containing a soluble fluoride compound is drunk, there are two ways in which it may act. First, the fluoride in the water may act directly on the tissues with which it comes in contact. These include the lips, teeth, tongue, and the mucous linings of the mouth, esophagus (gullet), stomach, and intestines. When the material reaches the stomach it will be mixed with and diluted by whatever happens to be in the stomach at the time, making a weaker and presumably less active mixture.

With strong solutions, such direct effects occur. Thus, when teeth are painted with a 2-percent solution of sodium fluoride, some of the fluoride combines with the surface of the tooth enamel, making a surface which is thought to be less subject to decay than is normal enamel. This is hard to prove, one way or the other, and there is difference of opinion as to how effective it is, if at all.

When the effects of a 2-percent solution are thus doubtful, it is not reasonable to expect much effect from a solution which is twenty thousand times as weak, namely the one-part-per-million strength which is being recommended for drinking. The 2-percent solution is far too poisonous to drink, and great care is taken so none is swallowed when it is used to paint the teeth.

There is no possibility that the teeth, once they are erupted, are beneficially affected by fluoridated water, and claims to this effect tend to cast doubt on the reliability of the methods used to support all the claimed benefits. Neither is there the remotest possibility that the other surfaces named, which are bathed by the fluoridated water, are appreciably affected at one part per million (ppm). In other words, when considering the effects of fluoridated water, the direct effects can be completely disregarded.

The other action of fluorides is essentially the same as that by which practically all the things we eat and drink affect our bodies. These are acted upon by the digestive juices, and portions of them are made suitable for absorption into the blood. Such portions are taken up by the blood, and the unusable portions pass on and out.

When the fluoride is consumed in solution, as in the case of fluoridated water, no digestion is needed, and it is almost completely absorbed into the blood. When it is consumed as a solid, and especially as a relatively insoluble solid such as calcium (lime) fluoride, bone meal, or fluorapatite (a complex compound of calcium, phosphorus, oxygen, and fluorine), smaller and variable amounts may actually be taken up by the blood.

Since the blood volume is fairly constant under normal conditions, it should be clear that the concentration in the blood at any time is the result of three factors: (a) how much remains from previous absorption, (b) how fast it is being absorbed, and (c) how fast it is being removed.

It should be clear that, since absorption of dissolved fluoride is almost complete, the amount which will be absorbed in a given time is related to how much fluoride is actually consumed during that period, and has no relationship to how much water was consumed along with the fluoride. In other words, the blood level of fluoride is related to the *dose* consumed, and is not controlled by the concentration in the water. The effect of one glass of water with ten parts of fluoride per million is exactly the same as the effect of ten glasses with one part per million, if consumed over the same period.

There are several ways in which fluoride is removed from the blood and carried from the body. Minute amounts pass back from the blood into the bowels and are eliminated. Small amounts are lost in perspiration. Tiny amounts are lost when teeth which contain fluoride are pulled. The chief way the body gets rid of fluoride is by means of the kidneys, which remove fluoride from the blood and put it out in the urine.

It has now been proved, however, that the amount put out by the kidneys is always less than what the body takes in. The result is that the amount of fluoride in the body increases continuously over the years. That is why it is called a "cumulative poison."

It should be clear that if the kidneys are defective in such a way that their power to put out fluoride is reduced, it will accumulate more rapidly in the body, and the type of poisoning which is caused by accumulation will come earlier and be more severe. And since kidney damage can be caused by fluoride, there can be a vicious circle by which kidney damage causes more fluoride retention, which in turn causes further kidney damage.

There are other ways by which fluoride can be removed from the blood without leaving the body. In fact, the only known damage which the fluoride can do while it is in the blood is to interfere with clotting. We suspect that there may be other effects, but we are not sure.

The function of the blood is to carry materials to the parts of the body where they are needed, and to carry away wastes, chiefly to the lungs and kidneys. It does the same thing with fluoride. In places where the fluoride in the tissue fluids is lower than in the blood, it passes out of the blood and becomes part of the fluid which bathes the body cells, and on which they depend for their life and activity. It is here that the effects of fluoride generally take place. The reverse process can also take place, whereby fluoride passes from the tissues and the tissue fluids back into the blood, to be carried elsewhere in the body, or to be eliminated by the kidneys. This occurs where the concentration in the tissues is high and that in the blood is low.

FLUORIDE STORAGE

The process by which fluoride goes from the blood into the tissues, and sometimes back, can go a step farther in the case of the bones, and to a slight extent in the teeth while they are being formed. This is because calcium fluoride is only slightly soluble.

The process by which bones become hard is by depositing solid lime salts in a soft-tissue foundation structure called the bone matrix, which determines the form and structure of the resulting bone. There is argument whether the lime salts are calcium phosphate or apatite and it is possible that they are both. In any case the chief constituents are calcium, phosphorus, and oxygen; and the depositing process depends on the amounts *and the proportions* of calcium and phosphorus in the fluids in and around the matrix at the time.

It happens that the solubility of calcium fluoride is almost the same as that of calcium phosphate, and if there is fluorine in the tissue fluids along with the calcium and phosphorus it will be included in the solid deposit which forms the solid bone.

We must remember, however, that bone tissue is living tissue, and these deposits are not permanent. They are constantly being torn down and rebuilt, from the same or new materials. Meanwhile these deposits act as a reservoir into which fluoride can go from the blood and tissue fluids when their fluoride content is high, and from which it can return when the content in the fluids is low.

The same sort of thing happens in the dentine of the teeth which is, in most respects, simply bone. It also happens in the enamel but here there is a difference. Once the tooth is formed and erupted the enamel has no circulation and is not subject to the building-up and tearing-down processes which go on in other tissues. The composition and structure are not further modified except by injury or disease.

There is argument as to how much storage of fluoride occurs in tissues other than bones and teeth, but if it occurs the amounts are relatively insignificant. It does occur where there are abnormal deposits of calcium in soft tissues other than bone matrix, and there is strong evidence that such deposits may be *caused* by fluoride. Fluoride in large amounts has recently been found in many kidney stones; but whether it plays a part in causing the stones has not yet been determined.

EFFECT ON ENZYMES

Almost all body processes are carried on by the action of chemical activators called enzymes. There are hundreds of these, each of which activates a particular stage of a larger transformation.

We all know that if you heat sugar sufficiently it burns and gives off more heat in the process. In burning, it combines with oxygen to form carbon dioxide and water and to liberate energy in the form of heat.

The body derives most of its energy from the oxidation of sugar and related substances, but it does it without heat, at body temperature. Appropriate enzymes carry the sugar through a series of transformations which liberate the energy without the fire. This is only one of the countless reactions which go on continuously in the body, each carried on by its own enzyme activators. The enzymes themselves are made by action of other enzymes, and the raw materials for all this come, of course, from what we eat.

It has long been established that fluorides interfere with the action of a great many enzymes. Not all enzymes are affected, of course, but the action when it occurs is very powerful and takes place at unbelievably low concentrations of fluoride. We must also remember that when any one stage of a particular action is stopped, the whole process stops.

Since fluoride interferes with the action of many enzymes, which are essential to many different body processes and functions, it follows that there is almost no limit to the kinds of trouble which could be caused by fluoride if the conditions were right. The only question is when and how often the various possible troubles actually do occur. At any rate it is not surprising that so many different symptoms are apparently caused by fluoride that those who want to think fluoride is harmless can say: "It couldn't cause so many symptoms. They are all just imaginary."

The fact remains that people "imagine" these troubles when they consume fluoride, and stop "imagining" when the fluoride is stopped, even when they don't know they are getting it or that it has been stopped.

ACUTE VS. CHRONIC POISONING

A large dose of fluoride taken at one time, or in quickly repeated divided doses, will kill. Information on the killing dose is limited, but the generally accepted lethal dose in the case of sodium fluoride is 4.5 grams. (A nickel weighs 5 grams.) People have died from one gram, and have lived after ten, if they vomited promptly.

Slightly smaller doses cause more or less violent illness, with recovery; and the recovery is quite complete if no further fluoride is taken. All but a very small remainder is eliminated within a few days, and the body has vast capacity for repair if given a fair chance.

Strangely, the body is less able to deal with minute daily doses of fluoride over a long period than with the same amount given in a single dose, so long as the single dose is not lethal. If you take two and a half grams of sodium fluoride and recover, the recovery is complete. But if you take a slightly smaller amount in doses providing one thousandth of a gram of fluorine a day for three years (the amount in about a quart of fluoridated water), there will be much more damage to many more parts of the body, and the damage will be permanent in the sense that the operation of important functions will have been so disturbed for so long that they can never again be completely normal.

CHRONIC FLUOROSIS

Fluorosis is the name applied to any type of chronic fluoride poisoning, and until recently it has been the only form which has concerned us in discussing the possible dangers of fluoride in drinking waters. All the talk about the hundreds of gallons you would have to drink at one time to get sick refers to acute poisoning, which isn't even under consideration. It is misleading to an uninformed public.

What is important is that the presence of tiny amounts of fluoride in the tissue fluids for long periods interferes with the proper growth, development and function of many parts of the body.

In the case of bone, for instance, the important thing is not the presence of fluorine in the crystals of lime salt. So far as is known, the crystals serve their purpose equally well with or without the fluorine. The important thing is that in the presence of fluoride the bone matrix is improperly formed and as a result the structure and even the form of the resulting bone are abnormal. And since later growth proceeds from the original patterns, abnormalities which were slight at first get farther and farther "out of line" as time goes on, even when the damaging agents are removed, much as a building with a crooked foundation may become more distorted as the building progresses.

In the case of bone, these changes eventually become so

severe that they can be shown by X-ray. In the case of other organs this is usually not possible, and all we know is that things just don't work as they should. We may know that the trouble *could* be caused by fluoride, but it is usually impossible to prove that it *is* so caused because most such troubles require years to develop and may not show up till long after the fluoride which caused them has been forgotten—if its presence was ever known in the first place.

HYPERSENSITIVITY

Most people can take aspirin freely, some take it much too freely, with little or no harm. Once in a long time, however, someone dies from a single aspirin tablet. There are many degrees and kinds of hypersensitivity which certain persons show toward substances which do not bother others. Some of these are well understood. Others we don't understand.

Recently it has become apparent that many people show hypersensitivity of one sort or another to fluoride. Dr. Waldbott has studied such reactions, and will discuss them in another chapter. However, we might consider why they should now be noticed whereas they have not been noticed where people have been using natural-fluoride water over a period of years.

One quite obvious reason is that it is easy to overlook something if you don't even know it exists and never look for it; but there is more to it than that. The fact is that the antidote to fluoride poisoning is an *excess* of calcium. Most waters which contain fluoride naturally are "hard" waters which contain much calcium. The fluoride thus brings with it its own antidote. When fluoride is added to a soft water, the situation is very different. The fluoride is consumed without the antidote, and it is to be expected that the results will differ from any which were common before. It is not, therefore, surprising that we are now finding a new disease, man-made by adding fluoride to drinking waters which lack the protective calcium.

The things we are finding in hypersensitive people develop quickly and are already being found. We can reasonably expect, however, that there will also be new forms, and more severe forms, of the slower types of damage which may not show up for many years. This is what we may reasonably expect if we go on fluoridating soft waters; but what type of damage we will find we can't even guess at this stage. When we find out, the damage will have been done.

Why Fluoridating Water

Supplies Is Dangerous

ADDITION of fluoride to the water must be sharply distinguished from the use of chemicals such as chlorine which are added for the purpose of purifying the water, or making it more palatable to the consumer. Fluoride is added for the purpose of acting on the bodies of consumers and altering their structure and function. The alleged purpose is to make their teeth more resistant to decay.

Thus, by definition, the fluoride is being used as a drug. Whether this does or does not constitute medication is a pointless quibble, used to confuse the essential point, namely, that the purpose of adding fluoride is to act on the consumer, not to purify the water.

Effects of Fluoride Depend on the Dose Consumed,
Not on Concentration in the Water

Effects of fluoride are not obtained by contact with the teeth.
When contact action is desired, the solution used is some 20,000
times as strong as is recommended for the water, and still it is
not too effective.

The action of fluoridated water is obtained while the teeth
are calcifying and before they erupt. The fluoride must be swallowed, absorbed into the blood, and carried to the tooth buds,
where it acts on the enamel-forming cells. These cells have no
way of knowing how much water was mixed with the fluoride
when it entered the stomach. They are influenced only by the
concentration in the blood. This depends on the amount of
fluoride absorbed, not on the amount in the water.

It is obvious that volume and concentration are of equal importance in determining dose. The effect of one glass of water
with ten parts* of fluoride per million is precisely the same as
the effect of ten glasses containing one part per million.

There is no dissent from the proposition that the effects of
fluoride are thus related to water consumption. That is why the
Public Health Service recommends that less fluoride be put in
the water in hot climates where water consumption is increased.
This compensates, in some degree, for differences in average
water consumption between, say, Phoenix, Arizona, and New
York, N. Y. It does nothing to compensate for the greater and
far more important differences between how much Johnny drinks
and how much Jimmy drinks in the same community.

DO PEOPLE DRINK APPROXIMATELY THE SAME AMOUNTS OF WATER?

It is common knowledge that some children habitually drink
many times as much water as others. It is also common knowledge that one child may be nursed, and later drink almost nothing but fresh milk and juices, and use canned vegetables and

* By weight.

soups. Such a child consumes little or no water from the public supply. Another child may be started on milk powder diluted with water, later drink almost nothing but water, use concentrated juices diluted with water, and use home-made soups and vegetables boiled in water. If the child happens to be a diabetic, he may drink water almost literally by the gallon.

It is clear that differences of ten to one in the habitual water consumption of different children are commonplace and that much larger differences can occur. Such differences can easily cancel out the difference between one part and ten parts per million of fluoride in the water supply in so far as the effect on different individuals is concerned.

EFFECTS OF DIETARY FLUORIDE FROM SOURCES OTHER THAN WATER

In determining fluoride dosage, one must consider all sources of fluoride intake and not merely what comes from the water. There is no such thing as a normal or average diet; at least, nobody eats it if there is. And even if there were, dietary fluoride would still differ as a result of fluoride differences in the same articles of food. As extreme examples, such foods as collard and buckwheat may contain no measurable fluoride or may contain as much as 9900 parts of fluoride per million, depending on the acidity of the soil and its fluoride content.[1]

FLUORIDE DOSAGE FROM THE WATER SUPPLY IS HIGHLY VARIABLE AND TOTALLY UNRELATED TO NEED FOR THE DRUG

No doctor in his right mind ever hands out a potent drug and says: "Take as much as you like. You are sure to get the right amount."

When fluoride is put in the water supply, no child gets the right dose of fluoride (whatever that may be) except the child who happens to drink the *right* amount of water. All others get more or less than intended, and often far more or far less. In either case there is nothing you can do. If he drinks too much, he has had too much. If he drinks too little, you don't dare supplement the dose because you can't know how much he has already had.

This inability to control dosage of water-borne fluoride is one of the reasons why the Public Health Service, if water is fluoridated, expects some 15 to 20 percent of children to have their teeth permanently disfigured by fluoride, while another large percent will fail to obtain any *benefit*.

Other Hazards in Using Water Supply as a Vehicle for Administering Fluoride

(1) When fluoride is prescribed on an individual basis, pure, drug-grade fluoride is used. This is both too scarce and too expensive to use in the water. There the commercial grade, plainly marked "for industrial use only," is used. If your druggist sold you such stuff as medicine, he would land in jail.

(2) Fluoride is a cumulative poison, slowly accumulating in the body with continued use. Some of its more serious effects may require twenty years or more to develop. Consequently, continued use after the time when its effects are desired involves unnecessary and useless hazard.

It is generally stated that the period when fluoride effects are desired is from birth to about 8 years of age. Adding fluoride to the water necessitates its use beyond this period and during years when continued use means increased danger.

(3) Adding fluoride to the water creates needless hazard to those unusually susceptible or unusually exposed to damage. These include: (a) those who drink unusual amounts of water, such as the diabetic, and those who do heavy work, or work under hot or dry conditions, with consequent large water loss from perspiration; (b) those with defective kidney function. Fluoride is largely excreted by the kidneys. When kidney function is impaired, fluoride retention is increased, and earlier and more serious poisoning results; (c) allergic persons, and those otherwise hypersensitive to fluoride; (d) undernourished and malnourished persons, and particularly those lacking adequate calcium. In this connection we should note that milk is an im-

portant source of calcium, and that those who drink little milk not only fail to obtain calcium but are likely to get more fluoride because of substituting water for milk; (e) those with occupational exposure to fluoride, and for whom any additional fluoride means increased hazard; (f) those living near industries which cause environmental fluoride pollution, and for whom any additional fluoride creates additional hazard.

NONMEDICAL DISADVANTAGES

Fluoridating an entire water supply to provide fluoride to children under eight is extravagantly wasteful. Only a fraction of one percent of the fluoride is used for the intended purpose. Of each $10,000 used for fluoridation, some $9,975 goes for such things as flushing toilets, washing clothes, and watering lawns, or for industrial use.

Addition of fluoride to the water supply may cause serious trouble with plumbing and equipment. Fluoridation has been discontinued on these grounds in several communities.

In 1951, there had been more experience with fluoridation in Wisconsin than in any other state. At that time Mr. H. E. Wirth, Assistant State Sanitary Engineer, Wisconsin State Board of Health, said:

> In addition to adulteration, excess impurities, and moisture content, there is the more difficult problem of incrustation control. The problem is common in hard waters, has been experienced, however, in soft waters as well, though not to as great a degree. Sodium fluoride when mixed with the water supply forms a precipitate with the calcium in the water, namely calcium fluoride, which has plugged injection lines, incrusted tanks and solution chambers. It was thought at first that softening of the supply used in make-up of the concentrated fluoride solution would control such occurrence. It has not in each and every installation. . . . It can be reported that great improvement and control of this factor has been accomplished through the use of sodium hexametaphosphate.[2]

We might add that sodium hexametaphosphate is not necessarily a desirable addition to the water supply.

Sometimes there has been serious difficulty in controlling the concentration of fluoride reaching the consumer. It is relatively easy to add the right amount of fluoride at the intake in relation to the amount of water pumped. After that, you trust to luck and anything can happen.

Pittsburgh, after seven months, had still been unable to reach the desired concentration as delivered at the taps. According to Public Works Director James Devlin, the city had been pumping more than enough chemical into the raw water, but not all of it was getting to the taps.[3]

In Morristown, New Jersey, after some 4 years of attempting to deliver 1.2 part per million, water from different taps was found to contain 0.0, 0.26, 0.39, 0.41, 0.05, 0.05 part per million, respectively.[4]

In Bauxite, Arkansas, on the other hand, three years after switching from water with high fluoride to a fluoride-free water, there was still enough fluoride in the system to cause mottled teeth in some who drank the water. This was attributed to incrustations in the pipes.[5]

MORAL ASPECTS

When a potentially dangerous substance such as fluoride is added to a public water supply, the burden should rest on those who add it to prove beyond reasonable doubt that it is safe for everyone. This has not been done. In fact, there is a strong reverse tendency to require incontrovertible proof of damage from opponents and to disregard or ignore presumptive evidence of danger.

What is more, the Public Health Service fully expects that from 15 to 20 percent of children who drink fluoridated water will get permanently and obviously disfigured teeth. Questionable or inconspicuous damage is *not* included in that figure, either.

The procedure when the so-called experiments at Newburgh and elsewhere were started was even more indefensible. The amount added to the water at Newburgh exceeded the allowable limit for a public water supply as set forth at that time by the federal government. Also, the experiments were in flagrant violation of the principles laid down at Nürnberg for protection of subjects of human experimentation.

But even if fluoridation were proved safe beyond reasonable doubt, it would still be in violation of the fundamental human right to determine what shall be done to one's own body. This is *the* most fundamental of the personal rights our Constitution was designed to protect. Without it, our other civil liberties are meaningless. It may not be abridged except when, and to the least extent, necessary to protect the equally important rights of others. Since tooth decay is noncontagious there are no grounds for protection of others from those who have it, or who may get it.

Whatever the courts may decide regarding the niceties of constitutional law, the moral issue is clear. Fluoridation violates the most sacred laws of God and man.

Safer, Cheaper, and More Effective Alternative Methods of Administering Fluoride Are Available

One method of obtaining the benefits of fluoride is direct application of fluoride to the surface of the erupted tooth (topical application). The fluoride combines with the enamel surface to produce a substance less soluble in acid than is normal enamel. This method was enthusiastically promoted by those who now urge fluoridation; but when it was decided to push fluoridation of water supplies, the enthusiasm for topical application disappeared. It is now disparaged, or dismissed as a poor substitute. In any event, there has always been real question as to the value of the method. It is certain that for many people it has proved wholly ineffective.

On the other hand, *any* method of administering fluoride by mouth in controlled dosage avoids most of the disadvantages and dangers inherent in use of water supply as a vehicle. There are literally dozens of possibilities, and of preparations on the market. The promoters of fluoridation in the Public Health Service and the American Dental Association decry and condemn all such methods as lacking *the vast background of experiment and experience* which they claim for fluoridation of water. There is, of course, no actual or theoretical basis for this claim. The experimental background for use of dietary fluoride is at least as impressive as that for water-borne fluoride.

To meet all such objections, however, let us outline a simple method for providing water-borne fluoride cheaply and in controlled dosage. The daily dose recommended by the Public Health Service is 1.0 milligram of fluoride per day. If a larger or smaller dose is desired, proportionate adjustment of the method is simple.

Any druggist can easily prepare a gallon of water containing 1.7 gram of sodium fluoride. If you give a child one teaspoonful of that mixture in his food or drink each day he will get a measured dose of 1.0 mg. of fluorine (fluoride ion) instead of whatever dose he would happen to get if you gave him fluoridated water. To avoid criticism of those who think water-borne fluoride is magic, you can give it in a glass of water.

The stock solution is relatively safe to have around, as medicines go. The entire gallon contains less than half the lethal dose of fluoride. The druggist may want to use 2.21 grams of sodium fluoride instead of 1.7 gram. If so, he is figuring in official teaspoonfuls. The child's dose will be measured in a real teaspoon, which is larger. One and seven-tenths gram is the right amount.

This method permits controlled dosage and controlled effects at least insofar as we can predict effects at all. In any case, the effects will be far and away less variable and uncertain than with fluoridated water. In addition:

It permits use of a drug-grade chemical.

It can be restricted to those people, and those years, when the effect is desired. This avoids the dangers of universal and continued use.

It is far cheaper than fluoridation. In fact, the fluoride for the gallon of water costs about two cents, and lasts over two years.

The most expensive items by far are the bottle (which can be reused) and the work of weighing out the fluoride. Even on individual prescription, the latter should not be prohibitive, and if done on a large scale it could be only a few cents.

Its greatest advantage, however, is that it is voluntary rather than compulsory; but that is exactly why health departments condemn it. The lengths to which they will go to prevent such alternatives to fluoridation were recently illustrated in New Jersey. We were told:

> A plan to distribute concentrated solutions of fluoride to families in Freehold, N. J., for individual use in their drinking water has been condemned by the state department of health [on grounds] that this method "has been rejected by qualified medical, dental and public health organizations as being ineffective in providing a proper dosage to minimize the occurrence of dental caries; and the possibility of unregulated intake in homes represents a potential hazard.[6]

Quite aside from the fact that the organizations did nothing of the sort, and with due regard for the possibility that any use of fluoride may be hazardous, it is still hard to see what could be less regulated than a child's use of drinking water. It is equally hard to accept such attacks as made in good faith.

There is, in fact, every evidence that the primary purpose of fluoridation is not directed against dental decay; and that the real desire is for a legal precedent for compulsory medication in noncommunicable disease. Health departments simply do not want any voluntary substitutes for the compulsory method, regardless of what advantages they may possess.

Convincing the Public That Fluoridation Is Safe

That should be the whole story. It is very simple, and quite conclusive. Effects of fluoride are determined by dosage. Dosage is determined *equally* by concentration and by volume consumed. Volume is highly variable and quite uncontrollable when fluoride is added to the water. Therefore, effects cannot then be controlled. Also, controllable methods are available.

Actually, it is far from being the whole story, since great numbers of reasonably intelligent people are convinced that the uncontrollable method is the better method. We need to ask: "How come?" Let us, therefore, look at the record.

THE MAGIC EFFECT OF ONE PART PER MILLION

A committee of three physicians studied fluoridation in 1953 for the St. Louis Medical Society.[7] In their report we find:

> For the fluoride ion, the ideal, or physiologic, dosage is approximately 1.0 mg. per day, which is achieved by the human utilization of drinking water and water used for cooking from a source containing an average concentration of 1 part of fluoride ion per million parts of water. This intake of fluoride is calculated as a proper addition to the small amount contained in various solid foods. The needs of the body for water are fixed by nature and, although habitual intakes of drinking water, or of substances dissolved in water, vary widely with the individual, the differences are not significant in altering importantly the effects upon the human body of these small quantities of fluorine.

Some people are so intimidated by arithmetic that at the first mention of numbers their minds go blank, and while in that condition they will accept the most outrageous statements without the quiver of a single brain cell. If, by any chance, that happened to you, go back and read the quotation again. When you do, remember that: (a) at one part per million, each liter of water contains 1 milligram of fluorine; (b) dose depends *equally* on concentration and volume; (c) there is no such thing as an average diet, and dietary fluoride is also variable; and (d) small differences *in concentration* are considered by the Public Health

Service to be "significant in altering importantly the effects" of fluorine.

In fact, H. T. Dean (of whom much more later) has said: [8]

> It is obvious that whatever effect the waters with relatively high fluoride content (over 2.0 ppm of F) have on dental caries is largely of academic interest; the resultant permanent disfigurement of many of the users far outweighs any advantage that might accrue from the standpoint of partial control of dental caries.

Also, the Public Health Service recommends reducing fluoride content of the water from 1.0 part per million to 0.6 part per million in hot climates. This also is a relatively small change as compared with individual differences in water consumption.

BASIC CONTRIBUTIONS OF F. J. McCLURE

The statement by the St. Louis committee cannot be said to stand on its own intellectual feet, and it is doubtful if the committee dreamed it up. On the other hand, no supporting evidence is offered, and no supporting authority is quoted. Where did it come from?

A clue may be found in a recent event.[9] Frank J. McClure,* of the National Institute of Dental Research in Washington, D. C., was given the Superior Service Award by former Secretary Oveta Culp Hobby of the Department of Health, Education and Welfare. In making the award, Secretary Hobby said: "Dr. McClure's classical studies on the non-dental effects of fluorides in humans have resulted in general acknowledgment that the addition of fluorides to drinking water is a safe public health procedure."

In September 1944, McClure told the American Association for the Advancement of Science that: [10]

> Children up to 12 years, also exposed to drinking water containing 1.0 ppm fluorine, will ingest via food and drink-

* A recent article gives McClure's degree as that of Ph.D.

ing water about 0.8-1.1 mg. fluorine daily, equal to about 0.05 mg. fluorine per Kg. bodyweight. Normal mixed diets alone usually average between 0.10-0.30 ppm fluorine, providing approximately 0.3-0.5 mg. fluorine daily, regardless of drinking-water consumption.

If you do a quick computation with these figures you learn some surprising facts: (a) normal diets contain between 3.5 and 6.6 pounds of food daily; (b) *children up to age 12 years* weigh between 35 and 48 lbs. and drink between 1.0 and 1.25 pints of water daily.

On the same occasion, Dr. McClure said:

> A reasonable estimate of the adult's drinking-water consumption in a temperate climate seems to be about 1200-1600 cc. (2.5-3.4 pints) daily.

This is particularly interesting since, in one of McClure's own published experiments,[11] the actual drinking-water consumption of five young men ranged from 1666 to 7666 cc. (3.5-16.2 pints). The higher figures were in a hot, moist environment but without activity. If the air had been dry, or with activity, the figures should have been much higher.

Also as regards children, and quite aside from the obvious absurdity of the figures given, there is evidence that McClure knew better. In 1943, he wrote: [12]

> Drinking water is a variable factor, especially among children, whose drinking habits are greatly influenced by muscular activity as well as by atmospheric temperature and humidity. It is also true of children's diets particularly that the requirement of water is largely met by preformed water in the food or by liquid food, particularly milk.

It is clear that what McClure told the A.A.A.S. was in direct conflict with facts commonly known, and known to McClure, himself. Yet it was published in the 1946 symposium on Dental Caries and Fluorine,[10] which serves as a prime source of *scientific* information for advocates of fluoridation.

His statements have been accepted at face value by the St. Louis committee and others whose minds go blank at the sight of figures. They form the *scientific proof* that variations in water consumption are negligible and that, with one part per million of fluoride in the water, everyone gets about one milligram of fluorine daily.

This, in turn, forms the basis of the belief that certain effects are produced by a concentration of one part per million and quite different effects by concentrations of 1.5 or 2.0 parts per million.

McCLURE'S "PROOFS" THAT FLUORINE FROM WATER CONTAINING ONE PART PER MILLION OF FLUORIDE CANNOT ACCUMULATE IN THE BODY

In November 1951 the Ad Hoc Committee of the National Research Council said: [13]

> Chronic fluorine intoxication characterized by bone, joint, and other tissue changes has been the cause of impaired skeletal function in Danish workmen exposed to fluoride dusts. . . . The presence of concentrations of fluorides in excess of 5 ppm in water supplies in certain parts of the world has been reported to have given rise to a number of cases of chronic fluorosis. . . . Fluorine-balance studies furnish additional evidence that the human body eliminates the major portion of food- and water-borne fluoride when the quantities ingested do not exceed 4.0 to 5.0 mg. of fluoride daily (McClure, 1951).

The reference is to McClure's chapter on Fluorine and Other Trace Elements in Nutrition in the AMA *Handbook of Nutrition.* It is doubtful whether the Ad Hoc Committee would have been so impressed if it had examined the actual reports of the experiments instead of reading what McClure said *about* them.

There were three of these experiments, two of which were

combined in a single report.[14] (1) He analyzed *pooled* specimens of urine from young men in various communities and compared the *concentration* of fluoride in the urine with that of the water in the respective communities. (2) While traveling, he compared fluoride concentration in his own urine with that of the water in seven places where he stopped.

He found *a remarkable relationship* between the concentrations in urine and water. From this he drew some even more remarkable conclusions. He concluded that:

> The presumed hazard of cumulative toxic bone fluorosis surrounding certain water-borne sources of fluorine in the United States is greatly reduced by this relationship.

Later, he claimed that:

> The data indicate that upward of 90 percent of water-borne fluoride (in concentrations of 0.5 to 4.5 ppm of fluoride) is eliminated in the daily urine of teen-age boys and young men.[15]

Both conclusions assume that the volume of water consumed and the volume of urine excreted are substantially the same. This, again, is contrary to common sense and common knowledge.

Combined water loss in feces, in sweat, from the lungs, and as *insensible* loss from the skin often far exceeds loss from the kidneys. If McClure's experiments proved anything at all (which is doubtful), they proved that only a small part of water-borne fluoride is excreted by the kidneys.

(3) The third experiment was on *fluoride balance* and was performed on conscientious objectors during the war. He measured fluoride intake when fluoride was given in various forms. He also measured total output in urine, feces, and sweat. From this he concluded that: [16]

> The elimination of absorbed fluorine via urine and sweat is practically complete when the quantities absorbed do not exceed 4.0-5.0 mg. daily.

This conclusion has been interpreted to mean that each part per million provides one milligram of fluoride daily. It is thus considered to confirm the conclusions from experiments (1) and (2) above. Thus is fallacy compounded on fallacy.

There are several interesting things about this last experiment. In the first place, the method for determining fluorine was one originated by Willard and Winter, and modified by Armstrong. But Armstrong, himself, has said:[17]

> As a matter of fact, in my experience, the determination of fluorine in urine and feces is extremely difficult if not impossible. The results are usually on the high side, more fluoride being found in the urine to which a definite amount of sodium fluoride has been added than is actually present. So, I have never been able to understand the results that McClure obtained which indicate the excretion of nearly 100 percent of the administered dose.

It is also interesting that McClure used Galesburg water, with 1.8 parts per million of fluoride, as one of his fluoride sources. But when his subjects drank as much Galesburg water as they wanted, it spoiled his experiment, and failed to prove what he wanted to prove. He says: [10]

> Daily fluoride intake in hot moist periods became quite excessive and variations from period to period were quite extreme.

Consequently, he restricted them to 1600 cubic centimeters of Galesburg water per day, after which they were required to use Urbana water, with only 0.3 part per million of fluoride. By doing this he was able to make the experiment come out right.*

He concluded:

> Exposure to domestic waters, such as Galesburg, Ill.,

* It should be noted that the Galesburg water had been used only for drinking. If it had been used also for cooking the effect would have been greater.

drinking water containing 1.8-1.9 parts per million fluorine or any drinking water which contributes an average of not more than 3.0-4.0 milligrams fluorine daily to the ingesta, is not liable to create endemic cumulative toxic fluorosis.[18]

Meanwhile, Dr. Wallace-Durbin has just reported some studies done at the University of California for the Atomic Energy Commission. She used radioactive fluorine as a *tracer* to determine what actually happened to fluoride which was fed to rats. She says: [19]

In McClure's balance studies on young adult men, he claimed that there was no storage of fluoride when daily intake was of the order of a few milligrams. The daily intake in his studies can be calculated as approximately 53 micrograms per kilogram, an amount nearly 100 times greater than was used in the tracer studies described here. The results of these studies, together with those of [others] who found that the skeletal fluoride content increased slowly with age on diets low in fluoride, indicate that apparently there is no level of fluoride intake below which storage ceases and excretion is complete, as was stated by McClure.

McCLURE'S STUDY OF BONE FRAGILITY

A series of newspaper articles was recently published by a State Health Department. It was called: Health Department Answers Questions on Fluoridation. One of the questions was: "Do fluorides make bones fragile?" The answer was: [20]

No. . . . A study of 4,000 high school boys and Army selectees from different parts of the country indicated that there is no relation between bone fracture and continuous exposure to water containing 2.0 parts per million—or even 4.0 or 5.0. The competent physicians who carefully examined these 4,000 young men could not find a single case of bone fragility caused by fluoride.

Thus is the importance of bone fluorosis disposed of.

If the young men had been examined, there would have been no way to detect bone fragility short of breaking bones to determine the force required, and then analyzing them for fluoride content. You just don't do things like that to people.

However, the *competent physicians* turn out to have been McClure, a biochemist; and the examinations were never done. The data for about one fourth of the subjects were copied from army records which had nothing to do with either bone fragility or fluorides. The other subjects were asked by McClure where they lived, and how many broken bones they had had. *That* was the examination.[21]

As part of another *experiment,* he recorded their height and weight, and for another, he took urine specimens, which he pooled. In some cases he measured the height and weight himself. In other cases, they measured each other. The only reason this is important is that, as regards reliability, what we were told is about *par for the course.*

About the study itself, however, there are aspects which deserve notice. In the first place, McClure, in his introduction, observes that sometimes fluorine makes bones fragile, and sometimes it makes them stronger. This would invalidate his statistical study in advance.

In the second place, two of the fluoride localities had only 0.2 part per million of fluoride in the water; while one of the nonfluoride places had 1.8 parts per million—almost twice what is recommended for water supplies.

SIGNIFICANCE OF McCLURE'S CONTRIBUTION

The reason all this is important, and the reason I have devoted so much space to it is that there are quite reliable reports, over a period of more than 40 years and from all over the world, of serious cumulative, chronic fluoride poisoning, especially of the teeth and skeletal structures. All these are lightly brushed aside on the basis of McClure's work, as having no applicability where there is only one part per million of fluoride in the water.

Another reason why McClure is important, and understanding of his reliability is needed, is that he wrote the section on "Non-dental Effects of Trace Quantities of Fluorine" in the *A.A.A.S. Symposium on Dental Caries and Fluorine,* which is, as we have said, a prime source book of authoritative information among fluoridators.

Even more important, perhaps, is the fact that when the American Medical Association Council on Foods and Nutrition was asked to study the safety of fluoridation, it had no one who knew anything about fluoride. It borrowed an expert from the Public Health Service—who turned out to be McClure.

He even wrote the chapter on "Fluorine and Other Trace Elements in Nutrition" for the second (1951) edition of the *AMA Handbook of Nutrition,* which turned out to be a propaganda piece for fluoridation. This led to many things, including AMA *endorsement* of fluoridation.

CONTRIBUTION OF JOHN W. KNUTSON

On January 17, 1952, John W. Knutson, D.D.S., Dr.P.H., Chief of the Division of Dental Health, Public Health Service, presented "The Case for Water Fluoridation," at Salem, Massachusetts. His talk was published,[22] and has been widely distributed as a reprint by the Public Health Service. It also has served as a primary source book for information on fluoridation in many quarters. In fact, the statement used by the state health department in newspaper articles mentioned above was taken almost verbatim from Knutson.

Among other things, Knutson says:

> We know that fluoride is toxic in excessive amounts [but] you would have to drink over 400 gallons of water containing 1.0 part per million at one sitting to receive a toxic dose. Such a large drink might kill you, of course, but water alone would do the job without any help from fluoride.

He cites McClure's article in the A.A.A.S. symposium as authority for this statement, but, for once, McClure is innocent.

I can find no statement remotely resembling this in McClure's article, nor even any statement as to the acute toxic dose of fluoride.

Also, however you may choose to define an acute toxic dose, it is presumably somewhat less than a lethal dose, which is what you would get from distillation of 400 gallons of fluoridated water. Moreover, no one has suggested that fluoridated water will cause acute toxicity, except, perhaps, in allergic persons.

Since the point at issue concerns chronic, cumulative poisoning and has nothing to do with acute toxicity, Dr. Knutson's remark may be written off as propaganda. Nevertheless, it is frequently and gleefully repeated.

Recently, an assistant professor of pharmacy wrote that it would take[23] over 1000 gallons of fluoridated water to give a lethal dose (4 grams) of sodium fluoride. Actually, the 1000 gallons would contain 8.4 grams of sodium fluoride, as any assistant professor of pharmacy should be able to figure out.

Knutson's article also says that:

> More than 3,000,000 Americans have lived all their lives in naturally fluoridated areas. In regions where water contains from 1.0 to 1.5 parts per million of natural fluoride, the natives are at least as healthy as you or I, and they have far better teeth. . . . There have been rumors (and these are not even half-truths) that the recommended fluoride concentration can cause, or contribute to the cause of any number of dire ailments, ranging from cancer and nephritis to discolored teeth. Not one speculation of this kind has ever been substantiated.

Notice the tone of ridicule in the term *dire ailments,* and its all-inclusive but wholly indefinite character. As to the items enumerated, the statement about discolored teeth is outright falsehood. They are frequently caused by the recommended concentration of fluoride. As to nephritis, of course it can't be caused by fluoride; but destructive changes in the kidney can. And as to cancer, the charge that cancer is caused by fluoride was originated in the Public Health Service and ascribed to opponents of fluoridation. More of that later.

As for the 3,000,000 Americans who have used fluoridated water all their lives, he doesn't say that they drank the water, but others have added that. We are told that they have drunk such water *all their lives,* or for *generations.*

This statement has been one of the most telling arguments in the case for fluoridation, and as anyone knows who knows anything about population movement and water-supply history in the United States, it simply can't be true.

Knutson cites as authority for his statement an article by Hill, Jelinek, and Blayney[24] which says that over 3,000,000 Americans *are being exposed to* such water. The parts about their being as healthy as you or I, Dr. Knutson made up out of his own head.

Knutson goes on to say:

> Some of the rumors linking fluoridation to disease have stemmed from the fact that fluoride can cause certain ailments. . . . When fluoride is present in concentrations of 12.0 parts per million or more there may be signs of undesirable changes in bone structure. Such situations, however, are invariably alike in one respect. When they do occur, it is always in communities where the drinking water contains at least 12 or 15 times the quantity recommended for controlled fluoridation.

Knutson cites six references in support of his statement. You would reasonably expect that they would support it. You would be wrong.[25-30]

In the first place, to call what they describe *signs of undesirable changes in bone structure* is, perhaps, the understatement of all time. In the second place, one of the references[31] tells that serious chronic poisoning was found in 12 percent of adults where the water contained only 1.2 parts per million of fluoride!

Chronic Fluoride Poisoning (Fluorosis)
of the Skeletal Structure

There are several quite different forms of chronic fluoride effect on bone, and the reasons why sometimes one is produced and sometimes another are poorly understood. In experiments on rabbits, Largent, Machle, and Ferneau[32] found gross bone changes in young animals at autopsy which could not be demonstrated by X-ray.

Sometimes there is increased calcium as shown by X-ray, resembling either osteopetrosis or a simple osteosclerosis. Sometimes there is loss of calcium and a condition resembling rickets or osteomalacia. Sometimes the findings are indistinguishable from rheumatoid arthritis or ankylosing spondylitis. There may, or may not, be abnormal deposits of calcium in the joints and supporting structures.

It might be well at this point to reiterate that the proponents' contention that certain effects are produced at higher concentrations but not at 1.0 part per million is contrary to all available evidence and to common sense. Effects of fluoride are dependent on many factors, not all of which are known, or perhaps even guessed. These include individual susceptibility and nutritional state, especially as regards calcium.

Insofar, however, as effect depends on amount of fluoride, it is amount consumed that matters. Any effect that occurs with any frequency at the higher concentrations which are found in water supplies will almost certainly be found in some individuals at 1.0 part per million.

Fluorosis was described in records of an outbreak subsequent to the eruption of Hekla, in Iceland, in 1845. Although many animals died of acute poisoning within a few weeks of this disturbance, most of them suffered no apparent trouble until the following year when symptoms of emaciation, decreased milk yield, weakness and impairment of the use of limbs, thickening of the joints, and development of exostoses of the long bones and jaws became apparent. Young animals suffered most. Mottling of the teeth also occurred.[33]

Since 1912, a similar disease has frequently been reported in cattle near factories producing superphosphate, hydrofluoric acid, glazed bricks, copper, aluminum, glass, and enamel.

In 1912, Bartolucci described a different manifestation of fluorine intoxication among cattle near a superphosphate factory in Italy. The cattle became thin, and the coat coarse and lifeless. The animals lay down and got up with difficulty, limped, and stood with curved, stiff backs and stiff hindquarters. Tender swellings appeared at the joints and, after four or five months, there was thickening of the ribs and the bones of the head and shoulders. Finally cachexia developed and the cattle had to be slaughtered. Bartolucci described the disease as conforming clinically to classical osteomalacia.[34]

Roholm, in his classic monograph on Fluorine Intoxication,[26] tells of producing both this type and the other main type of poisoning in experimental animals. He believed that this type does not occur in man. He was mistaken.

In 1940, Silva, Chapedi, and Pedace studied twenty-four such cases in a tuberculosis sanatorium in Argentina and had the rather rare opportunity to do autopsies and chemical analyses on two cases. Cases of chronic fluorine intoxication usually die of something else, somewhere else, and when no one is looking.

They concluded: [35]

> Que la fluorosis de tipo cronica padecida en la Republica Argentina por muchas decenas de miles de sus habitantes, es una anomalia calcico, no solo extendida a los dientes, sino a todo el esqueleto, caracterizada por una osteoporosis generalizada. (Chronic fluorosis presented by some 10,000 inhabitants of the Argentine Republic is an anomaly of calcium metabolism involving not only the teeth but in addition the entire osseous system and characterized by generalized osteoporosis.)

It should be noted that this condition was found in relatively young people, in contrast to the ensuing type which requires twenty years or more to become manifest at usual levels of fluoride intake, and in absence of impaired kidney function.

Along the same line, however, Lemmon, a pediatrician of Amarillo, Texas (with 3.9 parts per million of fluoride), reported:[36]

> Some of the [Amarillo] babies have more tendency to bowing of the legs, even in the face of constant antirachitic therapy, thus supporting the theory that toxic fluorides interfere with bone and dental metabolism.

A more generally recognized manifestation of chronic fluorine intoxication, however, is the one referred to by Knutson, and described in the six references he cites, as well as by numerous other authors. The descriptions are essentially alike. I shall quote the one by Shortt, *et al.*[27]

After describing the dental manifestations, he goes on to say:

> Affected children, apart from the dental condition noted, do not appear to suffer in any way from the intake of fluoride and there would appear to be an interval, extending from childhood to about 25 to 30 years of age, during which few or no ill-effects are exhibited. . . . About 30 years of age, however, the first symptoms of intoxication appear. This is evidenced by a recurrent general tingling sensation, in the limbs and over the body in general. Pain and stiffness next appear, especially in the lumbar region of the spine but also involving the dorsal and cervical regions.
>
> The stiffness increases until the entire spine, including the cervical region, appears to be one continuous column of bone, producing the condition of poker back. Such patients to turn the head must turn the whole body; in fact, the spine loses its flexibility almost entirely; accompanying the spinal disability, there is stiffness of various joints due to infiltration by bony material of the periarticular tissues, tendinous insertions of muscles and interosseous fasciae. This leads to various other disabilities such as loss of the power of squatting. The bony skeleton of the thorax is markedly affected and the ribs become rigidly fixed at their junctions

with the spine. This results in their complete inability to allow expansion of the cavity of the thorax and breathing becomes entirely abdominal, while the chest assumes a barrel-shaped outline flattened anteriorly. By the time this condition is reached, the individual is between 30 and 40 years of age and the later and final stages of the intoxication are imminent.

The patients exhibit a definite cachexia; there is loss of appetite and general emaciation. Symptoms of pressure on the spinal cord may appear due, as will be seen later, to bony encroachment on the spinal canal. There is loss of sphincter control in the later stages, and impotence is common. The patient is finally completely bed-ridden, while the mental powers are unimpaired. Death usually occurs due to intercurrent disease.

I have quoted this at length, partly because this is the condition to which Dr. Knutson referred as *signs of undesirable changes in bone structure;* and partly to emphasize the fact that, with usual levels of fluoride dosage and in absence of impaired kidney function, this is a disease which requires many years to develop, and that *children slated for toxic manifestation may show no signs of what is to come* except as regards their teeth.

Pandit, *et al.*[28] reported this same condition as occurring in 12 percent of adults in a place where there were only 1.2 parts per million of fluoride in the water. Most of the waters that produced it contained between one and three parts per million with some as low as 0.6 part per million, and none higher than 6.0 parts per million. Yet Knutson quoted them to support his statement that such things never occur with less than twelve to fifteen times the recommended level for fluoridation; and the Commission on Chronic Illness says: [37]

At levels of fluoride intake (8 ppm or more) changes occur in bone which may become evident by X-ray (bone fluorosis). However, storage of fluorides in the skeletal structure in the amounts considered here results in no functional disadvantage.

Prevalence of Nondental Chronic Fluorosis
in the United States

Chronic, cumulative fluorine intoxication has been produced in laboratory animals and its manifestations are well known. It has been recognized in men and animals exposed to fluoride in or from industry. It has been reported in those who drink fluoride-bearing waters in England, China, North Africa, South Africa, and South America; in fact, wherever it has been suspected and looked for. The natural question is: "Why does it not occur in the United States?"; and the obvious answer is: "It does."

Granted that the people described by Shortt, and by Pandit, were in India. Granted that the climate was hot, and large amounts of water may have been consumed. Many in this country also drink large amounts of water. It occurred most among the poorly nourished. Many in this country are poorly nourished, especially as regards calcium. It occurred more among manual workers than office workers. (The former drink more water.) In this country, also, we have manual workers.

Symptoms of fluoride poisoning are actually common in this country. The question is not at all whether they occur, but when and how often they are produced by fluoride.

Let's compare a recent newspaper account with the description quoted above. It says: [38]

> Rheumatoid spondylitis is a back disability that strikes men between the ages of 20 and 40. It is most prevalent in active athletic men and in the Second World War was responsible for 18 percent of all cases of chronic back-ache admitted to one of the larger hospitals.
>
> The disease is not new. The spine of a man who lived in 2900 B.C. showed evidence of spondylitis. The cause is unknown. . . . The disorder is suspected whenever a young man complains of persistent aching or stiffness in the lower back. . . .

Spondylitis begins as a rule in the sacroiliac region and, when allowed to progress, may extend along the entire spine to the neck. The surrounding supporting ligaments and muscles are involved, as well as the vertebrae.

When the nerve roots are affected, pain may extend into the legs, chest, shoulders, and neck. In time the normal curves disappear and the spine becomes more and more rigid until it is as stiff and straight as a poker.

There is no cure. . . . Rheumatoid spondylitis is a generalized disease.

The similarity is, of course, obvious; and while this does not prove them the same disease, it certainly does not prove they are not.

The same is true of other known conditions which can be caused or simulated by fluoride intoxication, such as osteomalacia, rickets, certain types of goiter, parathyroid disease, and hemophilia. All are common in the United States; and all may, at times, be caused by fluorine.

Why Is Fluorosis Not Generally Recognized in the United States?

It is frequently stated that systemic intoxication from water-borne fluoride has never been reported in the United States. This is not true. We have already mentioned the report by Lemmon. There is also the report by Linsman and McMurray of a man who died at the age of twenty-two with severe fluoride intoxication, demonstrated by X-ray and confirmed at autopsy and by chemical examination. (The patient also had a *severe degree of mottled enamel* caused by water containing 1.2 parts per million of fluorine.)[39]

It is true, however, that the reports are few. This is both the cause and the effect of the fact that physicians, by and large, are unaware that such a thing exists. It is hardly mentioned in the textbooks or in the medical literature. The number of articles in the X-ray literature, for example, in the past twenty years can be counted on the fingers of two hands (or possibly one).

Moreover, the articles which do describe it are not easily come by. I had to send to Oregon for Roholm's monograph, which is out of print. I sent to Stanford for the articles by Shortt and Pandit, and to the Surgeon General's library for the one by Silva, *et al*. Other articles are in the dental literature, the veterinary literature, etc., but not where physicians see them. The public-health literature, on the other hand, is devoted to proving that no such thing exists.

Another reason why fluorosis is not recognized is that physicians, like other people, are inclined to accept as normal the things seen frequently. This was illustrated by a study[40] conducted by the Public Health Service at Bartlett, Texas, in 1943. X-rays were made of Bartlett residents, and read by a competent radiologist at the Scott White Clinic in Texas. He called them all normal. They were then sent to a radiologist in New England. He found abnormal bone density in 11 percent of the people. The findings were normal for Texas, where fluoride waters are common, and quite abnormal in New England, where they are rare.

For this reason, a statement by the physicians of Colorado Springs that they never see abnormal findings traceable to fluoride in the water is wholly without significance.

When I was in Minnesota, where many people drink from fluoride-bearing wells and springs, we saw cases of osteomalacia which would not respond to therapy. Frequently we saw cases of ankylosing spondylitis. We saw calcified ligaments and periarticular structures. We saw calcified excrescences on the bones of the pelvis, which my chief told me were age change, but I couldn't help wondering why some people were so old at fifty while others weren't at ninety.

I don't know that these things were due to fluoride. I do know that they are seen much less frequently in Washington, where few people drink fluoride-bearing water. Moreover, since I have started questoning people I find that the cases I do see have lived where fluoride is common.

That brings up another reason why fluorosis is hard to recognize in this country. Americans, by and large, just don't stay put, and relatively few have used the same water for twenty years, much less forty; and of those who have, very few know how much, if any, fluoride it contained.

The only way to determine whether findings resembling fluorosis are actually due to fluoride is by chemical analysis of a sample of bone, for example. You aren't justified in doing this to people merely to satisfy your curiosity about something it is years too late to do anything about.

Further "Proofs" that Fluoride Is Harmless in the United States

Beyond question, the things that fluoride can do to people occur frequently in the United States. What we don't know is when or how often they are due to fluoride, and what, if any, other things can produce them. The Public Health Service, which should be interested in finding out, isn't. On the contrary, it is determined to prove that fluorosis does not exist. People must be convinced, at any cost, that 1.0 part per million is perfectly safe.

FURTHER CONTRIBUTIONS BY McCLURE

All the work by McClure of which I have spoken was designed to prove that fluoride *cannot* hurt anyone. It was also necessary to prove that it *does not* hurt anyone. In this connection, the reports by Shortt and by Pandit offered a specific danger which had to be met.

In 1946, McClure laid the groundwork for the defense when he said:[10]

> The interpretation [of the findings of Shortt and of Pandit] is made less certain by the observations of Day relative

to fluorosis in the Punjab areas of India. Day states that "No spinal disability or general disturbance of any kind other than the pronounced dental lesion were observed in any of the children."

Since this is in complete agreement with Shortt's statement, you might wonder where the doubt casting comes in. Few people, however, have seen Shortt's report, and McClure left out that part when he told about it.

McClure did better than that, however. Shortt had listed the bones in their order of frequency of involvement in adults. Most frequently involved were spine, pelvis, and ribs. *Least frequently involved were the carpal bones.* You will also remember that early fluoride damage of bone could not be demonstrated by X-ray in laboratory animals.[41]

These points should be remembered when reading McClure's statement to the Delaney Committee in 1952:[42]

> More recently we studied the development of the *carpal* bones of *children's* hands in Lubbock and in Amarillo, Tex. (4.0-5.0 parts per million fluorine in drinking water), versus Cumberland, Md. (no fluorine in drinking water). These data, based on about 1,800 X-rays, show us that fluorine in drinking water has not influenced calcification in these sensitive bones of children's hands. (Italics mine.)

He really wasn't taking *any* chances.

McClure also pointed out[43] that the people studied in India may have had subnormal living standards (they probably did have, but so have many in the U. S.), and that the hot climate may have led to heavy water consumption. (That also happens here.)

THE "STUDY" OF 32 FLUORIDE CITIES AND 32 NONFLUORIDE CITIES

Sooner or later, the wholly unsupported statement that over 3,000,000 Americans had been using fluoride water all their lives without harm was bound to run into trouble. Someone was likely to ask: "How do you know?"

To meet this hazard, the Public Health Service, in May 1954, published an article on Waterborne Fluorides and Mortality.[44] It compares death rates from five selected causes in 32 *fluoride cities* with 32 *nonfluoride cities*.

The causes of death selected were: heart disease, cancer, intra-cranial lesions, nephritis, and cirrhosis of the liver. No reason was offered for believing that the selected conditions might be related to fluoride, *or that others might not*. There was no recognition that people can be made sick by things that do not kill them; and you will remember that Shortt said the people with advanced fluorosis usually died of intercurrent disease.

There are other interesting things about this study. You would suppose that in studying influence of fluoride on death rate, you would study people who had consumed fluoride long enough to matter. This was not done.

Mortality statistics used were from 1949 and 1950. One of the fluoride cities was Grand Prairie, Texas. Its 1950 population was 14,594, but its 1940 population was only 1595. Obviously very few in the population had used Grand Prairie water for even ten years, much less twenty to forty. It should be equally obvious that the water supply for a city of 15,000 was not likely to be the same as the one that had served 1600 ten years before.

We must also remember that, as based on over-all U. S. death rates, out of each 1000 persons living in 1920, about 267 would be dead prior to 1950. In Texas City, Texas, therefore, with a 1920 population of 2509, only about 1839 were still living in 1949. Thus only 11 percent of the population had lived there as much as twenty-nine years prior to the *study*.

Other glaring examples are Snyder, Texas, and Elmhurst, Illinois, where only 13 percent and 17 percent respectively of the people studied had been in residence as much as thirty years. In fact, the median figure for the 32 cities was about 50 percent new people in the populations studied.

To make it worse, the source of water supply in almost every city had been changed or modified, not just once but often, in the course of thirty years. In addition, fluoride analyses were few and incomplete. Cities with multiple sources of water show analyses for only a few. Instances where the source has been constant were rare, and places where fluoride content over the years is known are practically nonexistent.

Quite aside from all this, even the facts which were known were grossly misrepresented in the article. When you examine the sources quoted by the article, accepting at face value the figures given, you find that some of the nonfluoride cities had far more fluoride than some of the fluoride cities; and that some of the fluoride cities had far less fluoride than they want to put in your water. You will remember that the same sort of thing was done in McClure's study of bone fragility.

It also seems strange that, with countless cities to select that actually are fluoride free, they chose cities with fluoride as nonfluoride cities.

We are forced to conclude that, however useful this study may be as window dressing, it leaves something to be desired as to scientific validity, and even as to good faith.

As a sidelight, I might mention that, in checking the bibliography of the article, I sent to the Iowa State Department of Health for its bulletin on Fluoride in Public Water Supplies in Iowa.[45] I was told they did not send it to anyone outside the state unless the person requesting it was vouched for by his own state dental health officer.

I asked the Medical School Library to get it for me. Twice they were sent something else instead. I finally secured it through the County Medical Society Library.

PREMATURE DEATH AND THE CANCER DODGE

It was no accident that cancer was one of the causes of death selected for study in the foregoing account. It was even dragged in again when a congressional committee was told about the study.[46] When asked what an intracranial lesion was, a Public Health Service physician said:

> Intracranial lesions in this particular case pertain to those instances where lesions are associated with what we call

neoplasms, forms of cancer; or other cerebral lesions which occur in the skull.

Maybe he just didn't know any better, but one wonders. In any case, and in terms of the effect produced, all the layman is likely to understand from that statement is that it has something to do with cancer.

There is no evidence one way or the other on the question whether fluorides can be carcinogenic. Yet fluoridators harp constantly on the theme that the *crack-pot* opponents even claim that fluoride causes cancer.

As I mentioned before, the whole story was started by the Public Health Service, partly to discredit all opposition, but also for a more urgent reason. It is primarily intended to discredit Alfred Taylor, and *to divert attention from the real significance of his findings.*

In connection with some studies on cancer-bearing strains of mice, Dr. Taylor, at the Biochemical Institute of the University of Texas, found that the death rate among mice given water containing 0.45 part per million of fluoride was consistently higher than among those given fluoride-free water. He considered his results tentative, but thought they had enough public-health significance to report to the State Department of Health.

He thought they would be interested. They were. A team of *experts* from the Public Health Service descended on him and his laboratory to discredit his findings.[47]

[The team] came to the conclusion that inasmuch as the [dry] food he was feeding his mice contained thirty to forty parts per million of fluoride that the ½ part per million in the drinking water could not conceivably have had much influence on his results.

Solely on these grounds, proponents have broadcast scurrilous attacks on Dr. Taylor, his work, and his competence. The *fact* of the higher death rate was completely ignored, together with the fact that both groups were using the fluoride-bearing chow, and that the only difference was in the water.

They also disregarded the well-known fact that fluorides occurring in food or minerals may be far less toxic than fluoride, and especially sodium fluoride, dissolved in water. Extent of the possible difference is shown in the report by Gershon-Cohen and McClendon[48] that diets containing 700 parts per million of fluorine as fluorapatite were not significantly more toxic than water containing one to two parts per million in solution.

Proponents made no attempt to repeat or check the experiments, but Dr. Taylor did. He used a larger number of mice, of a strain less susceptible to cancer. He used fluoride-free chow, and 1.0 part per million of fluoride instead of 0.45. He obtained substantially the same results as before, and about half the deaths were from causes other than cancer.[49]

He concluded that:

> The results show no change in the incidence of cancer, but rather indicate a shorter life span in the mice receiving the fluoridated water.

He estimated the amount of shortening at about 9 to 10 percent. This claim has never been refuted. In fact, *it isn't even mentioned.* Instead we prefer to talk about cancer.

More recently, Armstrong[50] tried further to discredit Taylor's work by undertaking to prove that fluoride does not accelerate development of cancer. He used a strain of mice so prone to cancer that they hardly live long enough for fluoride effects to occur. Then, instead of measuring the time till they died, which can be determined accurately, he measured the time till a diagnosis of cancer was made by examining the mice twice a week!

Proponents also obtained a statement from the President of the American Cancer Society, apparently unauthorized by the Society, that the Society does not think fluoride causes cancer. What that has to do with anything is anybody's guess, but it impresses people.[51]

THE BARTLETT-CAMERON STUDIES

In 1943, and again in 1953, the Public Health Service made what it likes to call *complete examinations* of people in Bartlett and Cameron, Texas. Again, there is far more in this than meets the eye.[52-55]

The Public Health Service says Bartlett water contains 8 parts per million of fluoride. The Texas[56] State Health Department says 6.6 parts per million. Neither says when, or what, changes have been made in the supply during the past thirty years. The U. S. Geological Survey doesn't mention Bartlett.

The Public Health Service says Cameron water contains 0.4 part per million. The supply, however, is from the Little River,[57] and such sources are notoriously variable in fluoride content. A single determination means absolutely nothing. Even from such a source as Lake Michigan, fluoride determinations on consecutive days vary by as much as fourfold at the same location. (Jan. 1, 1954, .12 part per million, Jan. 2, 1954, .03 part per million.)[58]

Actually, as in the case of other Public Health Service studies, they are not comparing a fluoride city with a nonfluoride city. Both are fluoride cities, and within a range where some Cameron people will ingest more water-borne fluoride than some in Bartlett. Consequently, fluoride effects will be present in both places, and any differences will be in degree rather than in kind.

Moreover, although all those studied had lived in their respective communities at least fifteen years, only eleven (14.5 percent) of those studied in Bartlett had been born there, or had lived there during the period of tooth and bone development. Consequently, when we are told that 11 to 12 percent of those studied in Bartlett showed evidence of osteosclerosis, it is somewhat misleading. Actually, at least 82 percent of those exposed to Bartlett water during the bone-forming period showed evidence of osteosclerosis.

The examinations included a test for syphilis, but did not include tests for such things as prolonged bleeding time, or disturbed thyroid function, which the Public Health Service knew might result from fluoride.[59] Neither did they examine the few who had been born in Bartlett for post-rachitic changes.

They did test for acid and alkaline phosphatase,[60] *when indicated*. They do not tell us what the indications were, how many people were so tested, or what was found.

We are told [61] that:

> When the data are reviewed critically, it is clear that the medical characteristics of the two groups, with the exception of dental fluorosis, do not differ more than would be expected of two comparable towns with or without an excess of fluoride in the water supply.

The trouble with that is that there are no data to review.

Instead of recording what was found, we are merely told how many people were classified as abnormal in various respects in the two communities. Neither the quantitative nor qualitative criteria of normality are given; and there is no possible basis for correlating actual findings with probable fluoride intake or with other pertinent factors such as duration of intake or age at exposure.

Even so, significant differences between Bartlett and Cameron are shown as judged by the authors' own criteria. These are casually brushed aside as having nothing to do with fluoride. This they call *reviewing the data critically*, but it is a bit hard to justify.

McClure knew in 1933[62] that abnormalities of the white blood cells were produced in rabbits fed fluoride by Schwyzer, who believed "these changes are due to irritation of the bone marrow" and who noted "a partial change of the yellow marrow into red." Both in 1943 and in 1953, "significantly" more abnormalities of the "neutrophilic" white cells were reported at Bartlett than at Cameron. The figures given indicate clearly that the differences were in morphology rather than in relative number. Yet we are told that:

> When viewed in the light of clinical experience, this finding does not suggest an association with fluoride intake.

One wonders why. One also wonders why about 45 percent of persons in *both* cities are recorded as having abnormalities of lymphocytic white cells. There is no explanation or comment.

Significant differences (P=0.05) in urine albumin and in cardiovascular conditions were similarly brushed aside, rightly or wrongly but certainly without adequate reason.

Another interesting, if not "significant," difference between the two cities was in the death rate. During the ten-year period between 1943 and 1953, the death rate among the subjects in Bartlett was 3.3 times as high as among the Cameron subjects. The authors explain this on the ground that

> the age distributions were similar but not exactly comparable, since in Bartlett they were predominantly older. The imbalance is particularly evident in the age group 70 and over. As a result, the difference between the age-corrected mortality rates is not significant by statistical analysis.

At that point things really become interesting, since, if you omit the older people from the figures, the difference is greater rather then less. If you limit the figures to those persons who were 55 or less in 1943, the death rate among the Bartlett subjects was almost *six* times as high as among the Cameron subjects.

I do not say that the difference was due to the higher fluoride. I do say that a sixfold difference in the death rate demands investigation before you can say that it was *not* due to a particular cause. Not only was there no such investigation; the fact of the higher rate and the need for explanation are concealed by a carefully worded equivocation.

Other major and quite interesting differences between the two communities will be discussed in Chapter 3, since they have to do with the dental effects of fluoride. Meanwhile, let us consider briefly the nonskeletal effects of fluoride.

Nonskeletal Effects of Fluoride

In commenting on the 1943 Bartlett-Cameron study, the National Research Council said:

> However, the greater incidence in the high fluoride group of a certain brittleness and blotching of the fingernails, of hypertrophic changes in the spine and pelvis, and of lenticular opacities (cataracts) of the eye, requires further epidemiological investigation.

Instead, we are told about the number of people showing "bone changes," which turns out to be something very different. The films from 1943 to 1953 were compared, and *bone changes* turns out to be the number of people whose findings had changed in the ten-year interval.

The 1953 report[63] makes no mention of the fingernails.* This becomes significant in light of the National Research Council comment together with the fact that Spira,[64] in 1943, had identified mottled nails (leuconychia) as an early sign of fluorosis. Of related interest is the fact that the same finding among the children in the Newburgh experiment has been dismissed as unrelated to fluoride.

The 1953 report does mention cataract, finding them in 10 percent of the subjects in Bartlett and 14 percent in Cameron. The difference is not considered significant, and no mention is made of the fact that both figures seem significantly high as compared with the general population in the same age group. In this connection we must remember that both Bartlett and Cameron are actually *fluoride cities*.

A finding of *decreased acuity of hearing* in 19 percent at Bartlett and 13 percent at Cameron also seems high, but is harder to interpret since the criteria used are unknown. How-

---

* The 1943 report was never published. We are only told about it.

ever, no attempt was made to segregate otosclerosis from other forms of deafness and, again, otosclerosis has been identified by Spira as resulting from, or at least closely associated with, fluoride poisoning.[65]

Spira has probably done, and published, more work on fluorosis than any man alive. Some of his conclusions are far-reaching and even a bit appalling. Many of them have never been confirmed by other investigators, but neither have they been refuted. His work is never mentioned by the fluoridators. Instead, he is subjected to personal vilification even more intense than that directed at Taylor. This is not an intelligent way of refuting unwelcome scientific findings. It might have been better to look for contrary evidence or to look for fallacies in his methods.

ANTI-ENZYMATIC ACTIONS OF FLUORIDE

The fact that extremely minute amounts of fluoride destroy or inactivate many different enzymes has long been known. This is highly significant when you consider that most of the body processes are carried out by means of enzymes.

In 1933, McClure devoted three and a half pages to reviewing work done on effects of fluoride on the fat-splitting enzyme, lipase, on carbohydrate enzymes, on glycolosis in muscle, on pepsin, and on urease. In the case of lipase, action on ethyl acetate *in vitro* was inhibited about 50 percent by one part in fifteen million of fluoride.[66]

In 1946, McClure said:

> Anti-enzymatic effects of trace quantities of fluorine cannot be disregarded. Studies by Robison and Rosenheim (1934), indicate an inhibitory effect on the action of bone phosphatase *in vitro* and suggest that anti-enzymatic effects of trace quantities of fluorine may modify calcification processes.[67]

This may explain the reference to phosphatase in the Bartlett-Cameron studies, but makes it no more meaningful.

By 1951, in the *AMA Handbook of Nutrition,* McClure states that the caries-reducing action of fluoride may be by anti-enzymatic action. Beyond that, he merely says:

> The effects of fluorine on enzymatic processes were recently reviewed thoroughly by Borei in connection with the report of his extensive studies on the inhibition by fluoride of oxidative processes in the cell.

and his reference to Borei's report omits the name of the publisher.

The whole affair is somewhat peculiar because McClure doesn't even mention his own quite extensive study of 1933[68]; while Borei, in the course of his monumental report on cellular oxidation and fermentation, pays only incidental attention to the action of fluoride on other processes. Borei says:[69]

> For further details of these phenomena, which lie in the sphere of clinical practice and are associated with the general physiological toxicity of fluorides, the reader is referred to the papers and reviews of McClure (1933), Roholm (1938), Mitchell (1942) and Hoffman and coworkers (1942).

and again:

> For further details and exhaustive bibliographies with respect to the general toxicity of fluorides towards animal and plant organisms, the reader is referred to the reviews by McClure (1933), Roholm (1937, 1938, 1939) and by Bernardi (1941).

Meanwhile, the significance of such work as that of Himwich and coworkers is completely disregarded. Himwich reported in 1941[70] that new-born animals have a special process for using carbohydrate which permits them to survive longer without oxygen than adults, and which is destroyed by fluoride.

Young rats (1 day old) are able to live in an atmosphere of nitrogen for 50 minutes. . . . Infant rats injected with fluoride and respiring air live for more than an hour. Litter mate controls, similarly injected with fluoride, but respiring nitrogen, survive approximately 5 minutes.

Similar results of varying magnitude were found in other animals. The implications regarding fluoridation are unknown, but we do know that fluoride passes the placental barrier, and facts lend credibility to the charge that stillbirths and neonatal mortality rates are higher where the water contains fluoride. We need to know. We also need to know what other body processes are unfavorably influenced by interference over shorter or longer periods with the normal action of body enzymes.

Conclusions Regarding the Safety of Fluoridation

On November 2, 1951, with help from McClure, the Council on Pharmacy and Chemistry and the Council on Foods and Nutrition of the American Medical Association reported that:

The Councils are unaware of any evidence that fluoridation of community water supplies up to a concentration of 1 ppm would lead to structural changes in the bones or to an increase in the incidence of fractures. The only difficulty so far revealed is a possible increase in the mottling of the tooth enamel. . . . Evidence of toxicity other than the effect on enamel has not been reported in communities where the water supply has several times this concentration. After considering the evidence available at this time, the Councils believe that the use of drinking water containing up to one part per million of fluoride is safe.

The Councils forgot to notice that the effects of fluoride are determined by dose rather than concentration. Moreover, and from what we have seen, if the Councils had actually *considered the evidence* instead of trustingly accepting what McClure said about the evidence, they would not have been unaware of dangers in fluoridation.

One also wonders whether the mere fact that they were unaware of danger was sufficient grounds for saying it was safe.

In any case, we may reasonably conclude that the *vast body of scientific evidence* proving the safety of fluoridation and stemming from the Public Health Service has far more political significance than scientific validity.

We may also suspect that when Knutson said:[22]

> Perhaps the most important single fact about fluoridation is that it will not harm any living thing or interfere with any industrial process,

he wasn't necessarily giving all the facts.

Our suspicions may well be intensified when we consider the dental aspects of fluoride intoxication.

Chronic Fluorosis

in Animals and Man

WHILE it is convenient to distinguish between "dental" and "systemic" effects of fluorine, we must not forget that any such distinction is arbitrary and cannot be sharply drawn. Fluorine, in the concentrations found in drinking waters, has no known effect on enamel of the erupted tooth. Its effects are on the cells of the tooth buds and on surrounding structures. These are actually systemic effects. Moreover, "dental health" is fully as dependent on the condition of the supporting structures of the tooth as on the integrity of the enamel. Position and alignment of the teeth and a correct bite are also important. All these things, as well as the enamel, dentine, and pulp of the tooth itself, may be adversely affected by fluorine in the water supply.

By far the best-known effect of chronic fluorine intoxication is the condition known as "mottled enamel" or "chronic dental fluorosis." It is generally believed to be the most sensitive indication of fluorine poisoning. However, this is because it is so much more obvious than other effects and *not* because it is produced at lower dosage.

CONTRIBUTIONS OF FREDERICK S. McKAY

The grand old man of mottled enamel is Frederick S. McKay, D.D.S. He was given the first research grant from the Research Fund of the American Dental Association to aid his study of this condition. We are generally told that mottled enamel was first described by G. V. Black, former Dean of Northwestern University Dental School, and McKay, as they found it at Colorado Springs, Colorado.

On December 29, 1941, McKay told the American Association for the Advancement of Science that:[1]

> The idea of studying this lesion with a view to determining its cause, had its origin as a research in dental science, in the Colorado Springs Dental Society in 1908.
>
> The existence of this lesion had long been recognized by the citizens and practitioners of that community, and the general opinion was that it was a condition that was peculiar to the community. . . . It had never been reported in the dental literature.

The original article by Black and McKay was published in 1916, shortly after Black's death. It was in *Dental Cosmos,* and was entitled: "Mottled Teeth: An Endemic Developmental Imperfection of the Enamel of the Teeth Heretofore Unknown in the Literature of Dentistry." This was followed in the same year by an article by McKay in four installments entitled, "An Investigation of Mottled Teeth," and with the same subtitle as the original article.[2]

All this is important because it gives us our first insight into the character of McKay's work. In the same article for which McKay claims priority, he quotes at length from a short but illuminating article on the same subject by J. M. Eager. This, also, was published in *Dental Cosmos* fourteen years before, in 1902.[3]

It is not uncommon to do what you think is original work, only to find that someone else has a prior report. However, few have the temerity to claim priority for an article which actually quotes from previous work.

Even so, there may have been some excuse for claims of originality in 1916. No classified index of dental literature was available till 1924. There was no such excuse when McKay reported to the American Association for the Advancement of Science in 1941. At that time he went on to say:

> It should also be noted that the first article in dental literature on this subject appeared in *Dental Cosmos* in 1916 under the joint authorship of Dr. Black and myself.
>
> A very brief reference to what was undoubtedly the same condition existing near Naples, Italy, by Dr. Eager of the U. S. Marine Service appeared in *Dental Cosmos*, March, 1902.

He forgot to mention that when he visited Italy in 1927, he had found that the condition there was *in fact* the same as at Colorado Springs. Neither did he mention that the condition at Colorado Springs had been reported in *Dental Items of Interest*, and in the *British Journal of Dental Science* by Dr. Fynn of Denver in 1910.[4]

Actually, there is every reason to believe that people have had *mottled enamel* as long as there have been people. What is more, we know that it has been in the dental literature as long as there has been dental literature.

THE HISTORY OF MOTTLED ENAMEL

Mottled enamel was not first found in Colorado. It was not new or unknown when found there. And it was not invented by McKay. It occurs all over the world, in both man and animals, wherever fluoride is consumed in toxic quantities.

In Iceland, it was called *gaddur;* in North Africa, *darmous;*

in England, *tooth-marks;* in Argentina, *dientes veteados.* In Italy,
it was called *denti scritti* or *denti neri* from its appearance, or
denti di Chiaie, from a locality where it was common. In this
country, it was called *Colorado brown-stain* or *Texas teeth,* as
well as *mottled enamel, dental atrophy,* or *dental erosion,* long
before McKay and longer before anyone knew that it had anything to do with fluorine.

There was nothing that can be called "dental literature" till
after 1839-40 when, within a year, the first dental school, the
first dental society, and the first dental magazine in the world
were all instituted in the United States. In fact, Oliver Wendell
Holmes tells us[5] that in 1820 there were probably not more than
100 dentists in the United States.

Yet an excellent description of mottled enamel is found in
Maury's Treatise on the Dental Art, translated from the German,
and published in Philadelphia in 1843.[6] Moreover, John Hunter,
in 1771, mentioned dark spots underlying an intact enamel surface which he considered a form of internal decay.[7] In 1845,
Blandin wrote:[8]

> Wooffendale* was the first to notice an anatomical pe-
> culiarity, which it seems to me I should mention here, not
> that I look upon it as a very rare thing, but because it is
> a fact which demands another interpretation than that which
> is given to it.

The anatomical peculiarity was one form of mottled enamel.

"DENTAL ATROPHY" AND "DENTAL EROSION"

Maury listed as erosion what we now know as mottled enamel
and referred to it as erosion or atrophy. Both names have been
used by many authors. He, like many others, listed three forms,
at least two of which are recognizable as what we now call
dental fluorosis. Maury also speaks of three varieties of what he
calls "decomposition of the enamel," two of which are also

* Wooffendale was the first formally educated dentist in the United
States.

manifestations of fluorosis which McKay has termed corrosion.[9]

There is vast confusion in terminology, and you can tell only by the description what each author meant by a given term. Maury used the term denudition for what everyone else has called abrasion. Black chose to apply the term erosion to what Hunter and almost everyone else has called denudition. Black then used the term atrophy to apply to what is now called hypoplasia, and which may be caused by fluorine or by various other factors. Black, however, was unaware that it had any connection with mottled enamel.[10]

An excellent description of mottled enamel by Meredith, in 1878, is worth quoting.[11] He used the term atrophy, then in general usage. This should be compared with McKay's account, made forty years later, for which he claimed priority.

> This word, meaning defective nourishment, although not strictly appropriate as applied to the disease we are about to consider, is probably more nearly correct than any technical name we have; but the plain English, tooth-marks, conveys the meaning in a plainer manner. . . . The term atrophy, in dentistry, is used to denote certain marks which form abrupt contrast with the general colour of the teeth, or which destroy the general evenness of the enamel by formation of little pits, indentations, or grooves on its surface.
>
> White, yellow, or brown spots of various sizes and irregular shapes may exist on the outer surfaces of the teeth; these do not interfere with the smoothness of the enamel, and although the teeth at these points are of soft structure and easily cut away, yet the places rarely decay if unmolested, on account of the lips keeping them constantly clean.*
>
> The little pits or depressions may be scattered here and there over the surface, or they may run together so as to form grooves. They may be shallow, affecting only the

---

* A better reason is that fluorosed teeth are actually less readily soluble in dilute acid than are normal teeth. The well-known antienzymatic action of fluoride may also play a part.

enamel, or deep, going through to the dentine. The incisors are the only teeth attacked in the great majority of cases, but occasionally others are also. Sometimes several of the teeth in one or both jaws may be so affected as to scarcely look like teeth, appearing as if they had been badly eaten and discolored by some corrosive agent.

The only treatment was to leave the teeth alone, or to extract them and supply artificial teeth.

This is a very complete account of mottled enamel as found by McKay at Colorado Springs and elsewhere, and by every subsequent observer. It should be compared, item by item, with McKay's account almost forty years later, for which he claimed priority.

McKay's chief contribution lay in exploiting the then new facilities for medical illustration. The early literature was illustrated by engravings and etchings, which give little idea of the actual appearance. And the fact is that the only accounts in the early literature which make any kind of sense were by men who had had personal experience with the condition.

McKay was able, for the first time, to show people who had never seen mottled enamel what it really looked like.

Significance of Mottled Enamel

Mottled enamel is generally considered the "first sign" of chronic fluoride intoxication. By this is meant the most obvious sign. It by no means follows that less obvious damage, or damage less readily traced to fluoride, may not occur in its absence. It is not even an early sign, since it does not usually appear until the toxic water has been in use for several years.

In the light of present knowledge, however, even the slightest mottling must be considered a sign of probable damage elsewhere. It is definite indication of toxic effect on the ameloblasts, and we have no reason to believe that other cells and functions are not at least as sensitive to damage as they. In fact, we have reason to believe that some may be far more sensitive.

ALL DENTAL STRUCTURES ARE AFFECTED, NOT JUST THE ENAMEL

In reporting on experimental dental fluorosis, Schour and Smith told the American Association for the Advancement of Science, in 1941, that:[12]

> In view of the multiple effects of fluorides upon tooth development (pigmentation, calcification, formation, eruption and attrition), the term "mottled enamel" is insufficient and should be replaced by "dental fluorosis." The latter indicates the etiologic factor and includes the dentine as well as the enamel.

We should also remember that while, to all intents and purposes, metabolism in the enamel ceases at the time of eruption, this is not the case with the dentine or the tooth pulp. There, the effects of fluoride can continue to increase so long as the tooth is vital.

EFFECTS ON TOOTH PULP

There may be a question whether effects of fluorine on dental pulp are due to damage during development, or in later life, or both. There can be no question but that serious damage does occur. Pulp stones and calcifications are produced, which often cause intractable toothache, loss of vitality of the teeth, and loss of teeth.

In the *Dental Practitioner*[13] for August 1933 are eight illustrations representing X-rays of slabs cut from fluorine damaged teeth, with normal controls for comparison. Pulp calcifications such as those shown are of frequent occurrence with even minute amounts of fluoride in the water. They are progressive with age. Diagnosis was confirmed by fluorine analysis, both of the pulp calcifications, and of the teeth themselves.

FLUORINE EFFECTS CAN OCCUR BEFORE BIRTH

It is generally true that even where there is rather severe mottling of permanent teeth, baby teeth are not affected. However, there have been many reports of definite mottling, and even severe mottling, of baby teeth. This can occur only before birth, from fluoride ingested by the mother and passed through the placenta to the fetus.

This was found in at least one place where water-borne fluoride was only 0.2 part per million.[14]

This lends importance to the work of Fleming and Greenfield at Yale. They found abnormal changes of striking degree in the pulp, the dentine, and the bone surrounding the teeth of newborn mice whose mothers had received sodium or calcium fluoride.[15]

It is also significant that Wallace-Durbin, in her tracer studies with radioactive fluorine, found highest concentrations of fluorine in the jaw bones and the incisor teeth, with slightly lesser amounts in the molar teeth and leg bones.[16]

Such studies contribute importantly to our knowledge, but also emphasize how much we do not know about the mechanisms by which damage occurs. The fact that damage does occur is, however, beyond question.

FLUORINE, CROOKED TEETH AND THE PUBLIC HEALTH SERVICE

Another long-recognized effect of fluorine is a tendency to cause the teeth to come in crooked. There is reason to believe that fluoridation will cause far more money to be spent on resulting orthodontist bills than would be saved even if the things we are promised about reduced tooth decay were true. There is also evidence that, in part at least, this may result from stunting of the growth of the jaws.

These things are hard to prove, however. Animal experiments do not necessarily apply to humans. No one can say how big a particular jaw would have been without fluoride. Crooked teeth do occur, both with and without fluoride.

One of the most telling bits of evidence is found in a study by the Public Health Service, and like so many other findings in the Public Health Service studies, it was buried and ignored.

A study of the teeth of adults was made in Colorado Springs, with 2.5 parts per million of fluoride, and Boulder, Colorado, with no fluoride. In the report is this statement:[17]

> Third molars have been excluded in all the data so far presented.
>
> In both populations the percentage of third molars which were decayed, missing, or filled was high, rising with age from 70 to nearly 100 percent at Boulder and from 50 to over 90 percent at Colorado Springs. About three quarters of all DMF third molars were missing in both groups. At Boulder 94 percent of third molar loss was reported as due to dental caries and about three percent as due to malposition of the teeth. At Colorado Springs about 36 percent of third molar loss was reportedly due to dental caries and about 62 percent to malposition of the teeth.

Nothing more is said, and there is no notice given to the fact that, taking the figures at face value, there were some nineteen times as many third molars lost because of malposition at Colorado Springs as at Boulder.*

Whatever the explanation, the difference seems too large to ignore. Moreover, we may be sure that there were many residents of Colorado Springs who had ingested no more fluoride than plenty of others would have received from water fluoridated at one part per million.

It should be remembered that third molar teeth lost because of malposition are usually unerupted and impacted, and their extraction is a far more formidable procedure than is the mere pulling of a decayed tooth. On the other hand, it is safe to assume that most of the third molars at Boulder had erupted or they would not have decayed.

It is possible, of course, that the entire account is misleading.

* 3% of ¾ of 100% = 2.25%   62% of ¾ of 90% = 41.85%   41.85 ÷ 2.25 = 18.6.

The purpose of the study was to prove that Boulder had more tooth decay than Colorado Springs. Studies designed to prove a point, rather than to ascertain facts and let the chips fall where they may, are notoriously unreliable. Bias is almost sure to creep in. Thus, in the present instance any error in the direction of decreased tooth loss from decay must necessarily be reflected in an equally false elevation of the figure for tooth loss from other causes. (Colorado Springs, 36 percent loss from decay, 62 percent from malposition.)

FLUORINE, PERIODONTAL DISEASE, AND THE BARTLETT-CAMERON STUDY

There are numerous reports in the literature that fluoride causes an increased incidence and severity of periodontal disease, with resultant loss of teeth. This is reported both in experimental animals and among people.

This fact lends added interest to certain findings in Bartlett (eight parts per million of fluoride) and Cameron (0.4 part per million) which were barely mentioned in the report.* In discussing the relative incidence of dental fluorosis in the two communities, the authors say:[18]

> Ten of 45 nonedentulous individuals in Bartlett, . . . and 1 of 64 in Cameron . . . had positive signs of fluorosis in 1953.

Otherwise, there was no mention of the fact that 40 percent of the people studied in Bartlett had lost *all* their teeth, whereas only 20 percent had done so in Cameron. This seems like a significant difference which might have been worthy of mention.

The difference, apparently, was not related to mottling. Only eleven Bartlett residents had lived there during the tooth-forming period, and ten people still had enough teeth to permit diagnosis of mottling. Granted that we don't know how many had developed mottled enamel elsewhere, there is still reason

---

* Other aspects of the Bartlett-Cameron study were discussed at length in Chapter 1.

to suspect that the teeth were lost from some effect of the fluoride produced *after* the teeth erupted.

In any case, and regardless of the time when the damage occurred, periodontal disease was far more common at Bartlett than at Cameron. We are told:

> Bartlett's DMF rate [combined total of decayed, missing and filled teeth per person] was lower than Cameron's in 1943 but higher in 1953. The latter was due principally to an increased number of missing teeth in Bartlett. At the end of the study period, 47 percent of the tooth loss in Bartlett and 25 percent in Cameron was attributed by the individuals themselves to periodontal disease.

It is interesting that, having thus used periodontal disease to explain away the differences in tooth loss, the authors tell us in their conclusions that there was no more periodontal disease in Bartlett that in Cameron. And the conclusions don't even mention tooth loss.

We are now told that the Bartlett-Cameron studies have disproved the absurd charges that water-borne fluoride causes periodontal disease!

PRACTICAL ASPECTS OF ENAMEL DAMAGE

We will remember that Meredith[19] said the discolored portions of the teeth were of soft structure and easily cut away. Other early observers noted that they are of chalky consistency, as well as appearance, and that the pits and grooves often develop long after eruption by a process of crumbling away of the enamel surface.

All this fits well with Black's histological observation, later confirmed by others, that the pathologic change is a lack of "cementing substance" between the enamel prisms. This may be very superficial, or may extend inward to the enamel-dentine junction. The spaces may or may not be filled later by a pigment which is termed "brownin."

Black, himself, tells us:[20]

When the teeth do decay, the frail condition of the enamel makes it extremely difficult to make good and effective fillings. For this reason many individuals will lose their teeth because of caries, though the number of carious cavities is fewer than elsewhere.

The same observation is repeated by McKay. It is confirmed by Boissevain, who said:[21]

Once a mottled tooth starts to decay, however, it deteriorates rapidly, as they are difficult to repair because of the brittle enamel and hard dentine.

Also, the Smiths reported a study of the durability of mottled teeth at St. David, Arizona, where fluoride in water supplies ranged from 1.6 to 4.0 parts per million. They say:[22]

There is ample evidence that mottled teeth, though they be somewhat more resistant to the onset of decay, are structurally weak, and that unfortunately when decay does set in the result is disastrous. . . .

Although only 33 percent of the children in the age group from 12 to 14 years showed any carious lesions, the percentage with carious teeth increased with age as was to be expected. Beyond the age of 21 years, there were relatively few individuals in which caries had not developed. That the result of the onset of caries was especially severe is reflected in the high percentage of all groups with extracted teeth. Caries once started evidently spreads rapidly. Steps taken to repair the cavities in many cases were unsuccessful, the tooth breaking away when attempts were made to anchor the fillings, so that extraction was the only course. That decay was widespread and repair unsuccessful among the young adults is shown by an incidence of more than 50 percent of false teeth in the age group 24 to 26 years. This high incidence of false teeth appeared in all subsequent age groups. Very rarely adults were found whose teeth, though mottled, were free from caries. It was the exception rather than the rule to find dentitions from which there had been no extractions because of inability to repair carious teeth successfully.

FURTHER CONTRIBUTIONS OF McKAY

McKay rarely mentions his most important contribution to our knowledge of mottled enamel. As far as I can determine, he was the first to point out that the yellow, brown and black stains which so often are found in mottled enamel are rarely, if ever, present when the teeth first erupt. They develop slowly over a period of years, often many years, in areas of what was originally an abnormal whiteness.

The white areas are, themselves, disfiguring. You can get a good idea of what they are like by sticking a tiny bit of paper to the front surface of an upper tooth. These are the spots which the State Dental Directors, assembled in Washington, D. C., in 1951, decided to describe as "eggshell white" rather than "chalky." [23] (They are now called "pearly white.")

As you can see, if you try it, this appearance contrasts sharply with the normal translucent appearance of normal teeth, and is little less disfiguring than the stain which comes later. Sometimes, in fact, the stain never appears even in severely mottled teeth. This happens more often in some localities than others. No one knows why, except that it does not seem to depend solely on fluoride concentration.

McKay's observations have since been amply confirmed by others, and by the published data of the Public Health Service.

THE INCIDENCE OF MOTTLED ENAMEL

Since the mid-thirties, McKay's activities have been limited largely to making appearances for the Public Health Service in support of fluoridation. His 1952 statement to the American Public Health Association was reported in *Public Health Re-*

ports, the official publication of the Public Health Service, as follows:[24]

> Fluorosis, even to an extremely disfiguring degree, can be produced when the fluorine content is two parts per million or more, but the caries experience rate may be and often is low. However, there are persons who use water with two parts per million of fluoride and higher with no visible fluorosis and a low caries experience rate.

This statement is more noteworthy for what it omits than for what it says. Also, for a vaguely implied support of the Public Health Service thesis that disfiguring mottling occurs *only* where there is more than two parts per million of fluoride.

At the time of McKay's investigations, fluoride content of the waters was neither known nor considered. In many instances, however, it was later determined, and extensive data were published by Boissevain in 1933.[25]

McKay forgot to tell the American Public Health Association that in every place he investigated in Colorado, where there was as much as 1 part per million of fluoride, from 85 to 100 percent of the children had mottled teeth. He did not mention that wherever there was as much as 0.2 part per million, more than 15 percent of the children had mottling. Neither did he say that he and John Frisch[26] found 91 percent of children to have mottled teeth at Salida, where the fluoride content was reported to be the same as at Joliet, Illinois, where only 25 percent mottling is reported.

It is true that some of the mottling was "of the milder forms," which the Public Health Service would classify as "questionable." It is also true that much of it was what the Public Health Service would classify as "a definite degree of mottling."

Moreover, in the case of "questionable fluorosis" the question is not whether damage exists, but whether it may be attributed to fluorine. This doubt is often resolved as the damage becomes more obvious with the passage of time. Teeth classified as "questionable" in childhood are often reclassified as "very mild" or worse with increasing age.

The Importance of Calcium

In 1952, Massler and Schour, of the University of Illinois College of Dentistry, studied the relationship of fluorosis to nutrition in Quarto (1.3 parts per million of fluorine) and Campagnano di Roma (3.5 parts per million), both in Italy. In both places "it was difficult to find an adult who did not have mottled enamel," and "percentage of moderately severe and severe degrees of mottling was higher in Quarto than in Campagnano in spite of the fact that the fluorine content of the water was lower."

They made extensive investigation, and attributed the difference to malnutrition, specifically to calcium deficiency. They say:[27]

> In contrast to the inconclusive data on the role of vitamin C and of iodine deficiencies in aggravating the effects of fluorides, there is general agreement in the literature that calcium deficiency does increase the severity of the manifestations of fluoride intoxication. . . . The data from this and other investigations suggest that malnourished infants and children, especially if deficient in calcium intake, may suffer from the effects of water containing fluorine while healthy children would remain unaffected.

You note that they said there was general agreement in the literature, but there is sharp disagreement from other sources. In October 1952, a State Dental Health Director was cross-examined in court regarding this article by Massler and Schour. He said:[28]

> H. Of course, I might add, too, that as long as we have enough calcium in the diet to form teeth, we will have enough calcium in the body or in the diet to form harder

teeth if fluorine is added to the water. You see, we do have
teeth in Chehalis—so we don't have a calcium deficiency.
We don't have a calcium deficiency if we have teeth. We
do have a calcium deficiency if there is not sufficient to
produce teeth and bones. We have humans born and raised
here with skeletal framework and with teeth, so if there was
fluorine in the water, if fluorine would be added to the
water, we know that those teeth would be harder, and by
being harder, they would be less susceptible to tooth decay.

❉   ❉   ❉

Q. In other words, are you trying to tell me if these experiments exist where this dietary deficiency showed that
fluoridation was dangerous, that it had to be in a place
where people didn't have any teeth?

H. I don't believe we could find a place where there was
a calcium deficient diet sufficient to produce any ill effects.

After all, he was a public official, testifying under oath as an
expert. Who can blame the court if it believed him?

H. T. Dean was less emphatic. When asked at the Delaney
hearings whether he felt that adverse consequences would occur
to any children no matter what their nutritional status, and no
matter what other variables might be present—he merely said:
"No." [29]

In any case, Dillon, in England, found that, *in vitro,* sodium
fluoride *reacts* with powdered tooth or bone, displacing phosphorus. Calcium fluoride, on the other hand, is merely absorbed
by the tooth or bone. The effect is reversible, and the calcium
fluoride is absorbed or released depending on concentration of
calcium fluoride in the solution.[30]

He also found that solubility of calcium fluoride is depressed
by the presence of tooth or bone.

He believes that a given concentration of water-borne fluoride
will have a larger or smaller "reactive" fraction depending on
how much calcium is also present, and that only the "reactive
fluoride" is toxic. Dillon has even devised a method for deter-

mining the reactive fraction analytically. He believes that he finds a closer relationship between toxicity and reactive fluoride concentration than with total concentration.

Obviously this is not the whole story, however. Since the joint action of calcium and fluorine takes place in the body tissues, calcium from all sources is important. Nevertheless, if the water, itself, contains enough calcium to provide protection, any deficiency in dietary calcium becomes less serious.

The relationships are highly complex, with many unknown variables. *A priori* judgments, based on theory, cannot be accepted without reservation. Nevertheless, the known "statistical" nature of equilibrium reactions between electrolytes, and our knowledge of equilibria within the body, would suggest that what occurs is, first of all, a suppression of ionization of calcium fluoride (thus driving fluoride ions out of solution) by an excess of calcium (the well-known "common ion effect").

In any case, we may be sure that the damage to any individual will be determined by the concentrations of fluorine and calcium, and perhaps other elements, in the tissues at the site and time of damage. These concentrations, in turn, are determined by many factors, of which the composition of the water is only one.

As we shall see, however, *it does not follow that the composition of the water is unimportant.*

Artificial Fluoridation

In 1939, Gerald J. Cox, then with the Mellon Institute, suggested that "the present trend toward removal of fluorine from water and food may need some reversal" and recommended that fluoride be added to water supplies as a means of preventing tooth decay.[31] One of the advantages he cited for this method of giving fluoride was that "the individual would be hard put to escape the treatment."

There could be no artificial fluoridation if proof of its safety were demanded in advance. There must be an *a priori* assumption of safety, for reasons which are readily apparent.

In 1948, H. T. Dean, Director of the National Institute of Dental Research, and arch-priest of fluoridation, wrote as follows:[32]

> A unique feature of endemic dental fluorosis is the long time interval between the operation of the causative factor, fluoride ingestion during the period of enamel formation, and the post-eruptive sign of the consequent effects. For example, the signs of dental fluorosis present in the superior permanent incisor of a twelve-year-old child merely point presumptively to a fluoride ingestion that occurred eight to eleven years previously.

Because of this, the original fluoridation "experiments" were scheduled to run ten to fifteen years before conclusions would be drawn. Instead, the Public Health Service dubbed them "conclusive," and embarked on wholesale promotion of fluoridation in 1951, at the end of six years and before mottled enamel had time to become apparent.

And it is obvious that even ten to fifteen years would be far too short a time in which to rule out systemic damage. We saw, in the previous chapter, that such damage may take forty years to become manifest.

THE "EVIDENCE" THAT ONE PART PER MILLION IS SAFE

As a matter of cold fact, there has been no serious attempt, and no intent, to determine what damage, if any, may be caused by artificial fluoridation. At the Delaney Hearings, Bruce Forsyth, Assistant Surgeon General and Chief Dental Officer of the Public Health Service, was asked:[33]

> Q. How much are they going to add in the way of fluoride?
> Forsyth: I believe the amount is up to 1 part of fluorine per million parts of water.
> Q. How was that figure arrived at?

F. I do not believe I can answer that question.

Q. Is there anyone else who can?

F. Dr. Dean?

Dean: That figure was arrived at on the basis of the study of the twenty-one cities and the earlier mottled enamel studies of what level of fluoride would give a marked protection against development of dental caries and still be low enough as not to develop any objectionable fluorosis. That is the result of plotting a curve on the twenty-one cities that hit about 1 part per million.

No such curve has ever been published. Another curve for the twenty-one cities, relating to the rate of decayed, missing and filled teeth to fluoride concentration has been published literally dozens of times, and all over the world, but not a curve for fluoride damage. If you try to draw such a curve, you have trouble. The data are so few, and so dispersed, that any line you draw is rather arbitrary, and you find little correlation between concentration and damage. The best you can do indicates a predicted value of about 17 percent "definite" mottling at one part per million. Whether this is "objectionable" depends, of course, on the point of view.

Let's get back to the main story, however. Dean further testified:[34]

In the 21 cities, we saw this difference of three to one between fluoride and fluoride-free populations. We set up a hypothesis, a dental caries fluorine hypothesis, and obviously the next step in scientific procedure would be to subject this hypothesis to experimental verification by adding fluoride to a fluoride-free water, and it is purely experimental verification of the hypothesis.

Q. Did you want to get experimental verification . . . of the fact that as far as you knew from your hypothesis no adverse physiological or medical consequences had ensued?

D. No; we were interested in observing whether or not we would get a reduction in dental caries, because we can see no difference between a fluoride ion in a natural water supply and one that is added.

Again, in the same hearings, Forsyth testified as follows:[35]

> Many of the questions raised during my appearance before your committee were based on the assumption that there may be a difference in the effects of water having natural versus added fluorides. In the field of chemistry there is no such thing as a natural or an "artificial" fluoride ion. All fluoride ions are the same no matter whence they come.

Now, of course all fluoride ions are alike. However, the conclusion that because this is so, all waters with a given concentration of fluoride will behave the same regardless of what else may be present, seems slightly overdrawn.

We are given another reason for believing that the physiologic effect of ionized fluorine is the same regardless of source, but that isn't very convincing either. We are told that McClure's experiments on fluoride excretion showed similar "excretion patterns" for all types of dietary fluoride, and that this proves that the physiological effects are the same.

We have seen, in Chapter 2, that these experiments are not to be taken at face value. But, even if they were, it would not necessarily follow that because fluoride excretion in two instances is similar, the actions prior to excretion are also similar.

"NATURAL" VS. "ARTIFICIAL" FLUORIDATION

As a matter of fact, the Public Health Service had long been aware that the composition of the water is important, and that the presence of other elements may alter the activity of fluorine. It was not till they needed *a priori* proof that added fluoride was as safe as fluoride occurring naturally that they started to scoff at the importance of water composition.

In 1936, Dean told the American Public Health Association:[36]

It may be reasonable to suppose that the mottled enamel index* will be found to depend entirely on the fluoride concentration of the drinking water; but it is possible, on the other hand, that other constituents of the water may have some influence on the activity of the fluoride. For this reason it appears that a careful survey of a community for chronic endemic dental fluorosis should include also, for the present at least, a chemical analysis of the water.

Such analyses were made and, in 1943, Dean told the American Water Works Association:[37]

Small amounts of fluoride are most frequently found in well waters, surface supplies being as a rule relatively free. Thus, if we compare the water of a relatively large number of cities selected at random we are very apt to have most of the fluoride waters in the "hard" water group and most of the "fluoride-free" waters in the soft water group.

Importance of this difference is indicated by a report by C. F. Deatherage to the American Association for the Advancement of Science, in 1941:[38]

In the east-central part of the state there is an interesting group of soft fluoride-bearing waters from another source. A shale formation . . . was eroded . . . and . . . distributed over the underlying limestone. This shale contained glauconite, a natural greensand, which softens the water percolating through it and also furnishes fluorides. It is these soft waters which cause the most severe mottled enamel.

And, since calcium and magnesium are the chief contributors to "hardness" in water, this might be expected from what we have already said about the importance of calcium.

---

* This is, of course, a measure of "community damage" and not of what happens to any individual.

FINDINGS IN THE TWENTY-ONE CITIES CANNOT APPLY
TO ARTIFICIAL FLUORIDATION

As we have seen, the "safety" found in fluoride cities is hardly such as to recommend it. Also, the safety of artificial fluoridation may well be even less so. Even so, the findings in the twenty-one cities are not even typical of fluoride cities in general.

It may have been mere happenstance, but most of the twenty-one cities were located in the limestone belt, where not only the water but also the milk and produce contain unusual amounts of calcium. In any case, except Colorado Springs, Maywood, Elgin, and the cities having less than 0.2 part per million, all the twenty-one had water supplies with more than 50 parts per million of calcium. Even the Lake Michigan supplies had about 33 parts per million.

This compares with: Atlanta, Ga.—2.4; Portland, Ore.—2.7; Boston—3.0; New York (Catskill)—4.5; Seattle—6.7; Scranton, Pa.—6.8; Philadelphia (Delaware)—12; Baltimore, and Richmond, Va.—14; New Orleans—15.[39]

It should be clear that waters which result from addition of sodium fluoride to waters such as these are very different, at least as to calcium content, from fluoride waters with upward of 50 parts per million of calcium.

This difference is highly significant. Joliet, Illinois, was said to have eleven times as much calcium, and half as much fluorine, in its water as Colorado Springs. We have every reason to believe that the elevenfold difference in calcium has far more influence than the twofold difference in fluorine in producing the dramatic difference in the incidence and severity of mottling which is reported in the two places.

Teeth Are Disfigured by One Part Per Million
of Water-borne Fluoride

We are told by the proponents of fluoridation that the mottling produced by one part per million of fluoride "has no esthetic significance." In 1948, F. A. Arnold, of the Public Health Service, wrote in the *Journal of the American Dental Association* that:[40]

> At these low concentrations dental fluorosis is no problem. Evidence of this was obtained at Aurora where although 15 percent of the children were classed as having fluorosis, only 5 percent of all the teeth and only about 0.4 percent of the anterior teeth showed even so much as the mildest forms of fluorosis. This minor amount of affection, which is noticeable only to a trained observer, is of no esthetic or public health significance.

The reference, again, is to the study of the twenty-one cities,[41,42] and Arnold, being one of its authors, should have known better. If you include the cuspids as well as the incisors as "front teeth," the 633 children at Aurora had 7496 front teeth. Four-tenths percent of this number would be only thirty teeth. Actually there were almost twice that number of *incisors alone* that were reported as mottled.

Dean, another of the authors, made the story still better when he testified under oath to the Delaney Committee:[43]

> Q. Well, these [mottled] teeth could be front teeth, too, could they not?
> Dean: No, they would invariably be the second bicuspid or molar teeth, calcified at a later date.

At the same hearing, Dean testified that from one part per million of fluoride, there would be no "objectionable"* mottling,

---

* The use of this word will be discussed later.

that the resulting mottling could not be noticed, that there would be no dull white opacity or brown stain, and that he would not recommend any fluoridation which would produce any "mild" fluorosis.[44]

Now, as a matter of fact, in the twenty-one cities, every city with more than 0.3 part per million of fluoride had some children with fluorosis classified as "mild" by Dean's own classification.[45] Also, every city but one had children classified as "very mild." Moreover, "mild" fluorosis *frequently* develops brown stain, and "very mild" sometimes does.

Elsewhere, I have published a detailed analysis of Dean's own published works and data, proving that these statements of the fluoridators are not true.[46] In the *Dental Practitioner*[13] for August 1953 is a picture of teeth with "very mild" mottling, caused by water containing considerably less than one part per million of fluoride.

The owner was born at Salida, Colorado, reported as having 0.6 part per million at about that time, but later as having 1.3.[47] At age six months, she moved to Westminster. Fluoride content of the well she used is unknown but, in general, wells in this region are reported to have on the order of ½ part per million of fluoride.

Another photograph in the *Dental Practitioner* shows teeth that would be classified as "mild" mottling. These teeth were calcified in Denver, where there are several sources of water which range from 0.1 to 0.9 part per million. Boissevain[48] found 0.5 in the mixture at the time this man was a child. And Denver has recently considered fluoridating its water.

Cases such as these are not exceptional. In fact, if we examine the data from the Public Health Service studies, instead of believing what we are told about the studies, we discover that in almost every place where any considerable number of people were using water with measurable amounts of fluoride, at least some cases such as these, and often much worse, were found.

The Strange Story of the Twenty-one Cities

It is not enough to prove that the things we are told about the disfiguring effects of fluoride are not true. We need to examine the evidence which has led countless numbers of people to unsound conclusions.

The misrepresentations by Arnold and Dean do not alter the fact that, at Aurora, there was a rather remarkable freedom from mottling of the anterior teeth.

EFFECT OF THE AGE AT WHICH DAMAGE WAS PRODUCED

Almost without exception, every observer of mottled enamel has reported that the teeth most often and most severely affected are the upper front teeth. Yet we are told by the proponents of fluoridation that at one part per million this is not true. There should be an explanation having nothing to do with one part per million, since the effect on any individual is related to dosage, not concentration.

There is an explanation, and it is fairly obvious when the underlying facts are considered. Many of the earlier reports commented that, since the enamel is fully formed when the tooth erupts, any structural damage must occur before eruption, while the tooth is calcifying.

Schour and Smith[49] found that, within an hour of administration of fluoride, effect on the enamel-forming cells could be seen under the microscope. Both in rats, and a human, when injections were given a few days apart, the portions of enamel and dentine which were calcifying at the time of injection could later be identified by ringlike defects like the rings in a tree trunk.

The importance of all this becomes clear when we consider that there are three groups of permanent teeth as regards time of calcification. First molars and central incisors start to calcify at birth, followed shortly by the other incisors and the cuspids. The second group consists of bicuspids and second molars, which start to calcify at about age three. The third group is composed of wisdom teeth, which calcify at a much later date.[50]

McKay was the first to point out that when children are born in a nonendemic area, and move to an endemic region after the age of three or four, there is no mottling of the front teeth, and only the second and third groups are affected. The same thing happened when a community changed from a fluoride-free to a fluoride-bearing water supply. Of course, the converse occurred when the change was in the other direction.

It is obvious that these things must be true. They have been found so, repeatedly and consistently, both by McKay and by others. When, therefore, the Public Health Service wanted to prove that only back teeth are affected at one part per million, it was not at all hard to do so.

THE CASE OF AURORA

Aurora was one of the cities in McClure's inadequate studies on fluoride excretion, and fluoride effects on bones and growth. It is also the "fluoride city" selected for comparison with Grand Rapids and Muskegon in the Grand Rapids "experiment" on fluoridation.

But, what was more important, and what concerns us here, is that it was the city selected to prove that fluoride at one part per million affects chiefly the back teeth.

Prior to the date of the study, in 1939, Aurora used water from thirteen different wells. The proportionate contribution of each well to the supply varied greatly, and is largely unknown. The following data are taken from the water history, included in fine print in the original article.[51]

The children studied were born in 1925, 1926, and 1927. Wells eleven and twelve were added when their front teeth were partially or completely calcified, but before bicuspids and second molars calcified.

Well 12a was added after the latter teeth were calcified, but before the analyses. The analyses were done in 1939, and included only a mixture of waters from wells 11, 12, and 12a. These averaged 1.2 parts per million, with a low of 1.1 and a high of 1.3.

TABLE 1

Well Number	Date Drilled	Fluoride in ppm	Date Abandoned
1	1891	?	Not given
2	1892	?	Not given
3	1893	?	Not given
4	1895	?	Not given
5	1910	?	Not given*
6	1915	0.5	Still in use
7	1916	0.7	Still in use
8	1916	1.3	Still in use
9	1923	1.3	Still in use
10	1923	1.1	Still in use
11	1928	?	Still in use
12	1929	?	Still in use
12a	1936	?	Still in use

The only other known analyses of Aurora water near that time were one in 1936[52] and another in 1940.[53] Both found 1.0 part per million of fluorine, but there is no mention of the source of either sample, nor of what wells were represented. It is not even clear whether the 1936 sample was taken before or after well No. 12a was drilled.

Otherwise, the facts are all there in the fine print, for any and all to see. However, it is so much easier to assume what is implied, or to believe what you are told, than to study page after page of fine print.

And even to read the fine print is not enough, because in the same water history of Aurora where the above facts are given, Dean concludes:

* Well No. 5 is reported to have been out of use from 1935 to 1939 and for an unstated prior period. It was repaired and returned to use in 1940. No figures for fluoride content, either before or after repair, are given.

From the standpoint of a population exposed for a long period of time to a water supply containing small amounts of fluorides, Aurora appears to offer many advantages for epidemiological study. Since 1898 the public water supply has been obtained from wells *into* the Cambrian "Potsdam" sandstone. (Italics mine.)

What those advantages were is fairly obvious, and they had nothing to do with an unchanged water supply, of known fluoride concentration, "during the period concomitant with the life of the group examined."

He fails to mention that the "wells into the Cambrian sandstone" also passed through, and received varying amounts of water from, the water-bearing Niagaran limestone and St. Peter sandstone. And *since that time* he has settled for telling people that Aurora has had the same *type* of water supply for over fifty years.

It is not hard to see why Aurora had only about half as much fluorosis as either Maywood or East Moline which are listed as having the same amount of fluoride. Neither is it hard to understand why the front teeth, calcified before 1928-29, showed less fluorosis than the back teeth which were calcified later.

AURORA HAS LOTS OF COMPANY

Under cross-examination before the Delaney Committee, Dean[54] explained the embarrassingly high incidence of mottled enamel at Maywood (1.2 parts per million) and at Marion (0.4 part per million) on grounds that there had been changes in their water supplies during the lifetime of the group examined. This, however, has not prevented their being retained as part of the study.

Moreover, Dean didn't remember, or at least neglected to mention, that similar changes had occurred at Galesburg, Elmhurst, Aurora, East Moline, Joliet, and Elgin, and probably at Lima. The "twenty-one cities," therefore, boil down to twelve.

Of these, Colorado Springs has 2.6 parts per million, nine have 0.2 part per million or less, and in the whole critical range between we have only Kewanee, with 0.9, and Pueblo, with 0.6.

It seems clear, therefore, that when Dean said the findings at Maywood and Marion didn't mean anything, he should have included the whole study.

DEAN'S "REQUISITES FOR QUANTITATIVE STUDY" OF FLUOROSIS

It is hard to ascribe these things to happenstance. In 1936, Dean wrote:[55]

> Because of possible changes in the fluoride content of water supplies, it is obvious that an attempt to correlate clinical observations with a single fluoride determination of a municipal water associated with endemic mottled enamel introduces the possibility of questionable correlation. In respect to water from deep wells, the fact that the mineral content usually varies within comparatively narrow limits might be misleading until it has been definitely ascertained that there have been no changes in the physical set-up of the water supply during the lifetime of the children. Hence the amount of fluoride in a water sample taken at the time of the clinical examination may mean little unless a complete history of the water supply concomitant with the life of the children examined, has been obtained.

In the same article he gave water histories for ten of the cities he had studied, and listed six of them as lacking the "requisites for quantitative valuation." This has not stood in the way of his using them.

He used data from five of these six cities in an article the following year. Again, in 1942, he used them in a chart to prove that the "community index of dental fluorosis" (his then new "weighted average index") was directly related to the fluoride content of the water.[56]

On October 20, 1955, Dean presented this chart in evidence

when testifying before the California Public Utilities Commission. Under cross-examination he was forced to admit that the chart contained the data he had listed as lacking the requisites for quantitative evaluation, and that he had known the data were worthless when he made the chart. It also contains the data from Marion, Ohio, which Dean told the Delaney Committee didn't mean anything, and from Elmhurst, Joliet, Aurora, Elgin, and Lima, which we know are also worthless.

In spite of all this, in the January 1956 issue of the *Journal of the American Dental Association* was an article by Dean, in which he used the same chart to prove that "a 1.0 ppm of fluoride (F.) concentration was well within the limits of public health safety."

Even more interesting is the fact that one of the six was Galesburg, Illinois. In spite of this, Galesburg was one of six cities used to prove, and itself provided the final proof, that fluoride protects against tooth decay even in absence of visible mottling. Galesburg was also one of the four cities on which the promised figure of 60 to 65 percent less tooth decay is based.

When, in addition, Galesburg turns up as one of the twenty-one cities, we may be justified in wondering whether it possesses other advantages which more than offset the fact that it failed to meet Dean's own requisites for reliability.

We already know that it had 57 parts per million of calcium, and have noted the resulting advantage. It seems possible, however, that in our discussion of fluoride and dental decay, we may find additional reasons for the persistent use of data from Galesburg.

Fluorine and Dental Caries

In the matter of fluorine intoxication, including dental fluorosis, the main facts are fairly clear, once you dig them out. When we come to the subject of fluorine and tooth decay, we enter Never-Never-Land, with no reliable landmarks. It seems fairly clear that decay behaves differently, and has different consequences, in fluorosed than in non-fluorosed teeth. Beyond that, all bets are off.

Aside from deliberate muddying of the waters, here and there, there is a basic reason. There is no way to measure either amount or activity of decay. You can look in two mouths and say, sometimes with considerable certainty, that one has more or worse decay than the other. There is, however, no number that you can attach to that difference that has any possible meaning.

Consequently there can be no meaningful statistics of tooth decay, and all the talk about 60 percent reductions, or any other reduction, in tooth decay is just plain nonsense.

In spite of the fact there can be no unit for measurement of tooth decay that means anything, and no way to apply it if there were, the Public Health Service invented one. It is called the DMF rate, and consists of the combined sum of decayed, missing and filled teeth per person, or per hundred people.

SIGNIFICANCE OF THE DMF RATE

In this total of decayed, missing and filled teeth, which is called the DMF rate, the tiniest cavity counts the same as a tooth completely destroyed, and a cavity filled fifty years ago counts the same as active disease. It is as silly and pointless as children counting their coins without regard to denomination, to see who has the most money.

When we were taught, in grade school, that you cannot add dissimilar things, or even different units of the same thing, it was not because of any narrow-minded prejudice of the teacher. It was simply that when you do, the answer you get doesn't mean anything. The five you get by adding four boys and one bicycle has nothing to do with the five you get by adding one boy and four bicycles, and neither is five of anything.

Neither can you add one foot and four inches and get five of anything. It is either 16 inches, or 1⅓ feet. Moreover, you don't solve the difficulty by calling your "answers" five boy-bicycles or five foot-inches.

It should not be necessary thus to belabor the point, but apparently it is. People are spending good time and public money making expensive and meaningless surveys of DMF rates, and other people pay reverent attention to nonsense based on the resulting nonsense.

Such things don't work in mathematics, in physics, in chemistry, or anywhere else. They don't work any better in dentistry, or in statistics, even when the methods are invented and exploited by the government.

THE "INCIDENCE" RATE

The fallacy of the DMF rate is avoided by using incidence rate—the percentage of people who have, or have had, tooth decay, as against the percentage who have not, and never have had. It is reasonable to assume that those who have had no decay have some measure of immunity, and it is reasonable to calculate the percentage who have shown such immunity. It is clear that the longer a person goes without decay, the more real the immunity is likely to prove. Consequently, such studies mean most in adults, and have little or no meaning in children.

Studies done by Ockerse, in South Africa, were based on incidence rates and, consequently, merit respectful notice as compared with DMF studies in this country and elsewhere.

Even here, we run into the problem of deciding "when is decay." This is not important in daily life. If the dentist can't tell whether you have a cavity, you can wait and see.

If, however, you must decide right now, for statistical purposes, whether someone does or does not have tooth decay, the margin of error is unbelievable. I have discussed this at length elsewhere[57] and will merely say, here, that it is so large that 60-percent reductions would be lost in the experimental error.

CALCIUM ALSO IMPORTANT IN TOOTH DECAY

Agnew and Agnew, in China,[58] and Weaver, in England,[59] found no relationship between fluorine and tooth decay. Ockerse, in South Africa,[60] found some correlation, but dispersion was so great that cities with high fluorine might have many times the incidence of decay of cities without.

If, on the other hand, he made a multiple correlation of tooth decay against combined factors of fluorine, hardness, and hydrogen-ion concentration, he found almost perfect correlation in *districts*. In *communities* the correlation was considerably less perfect, and the pH less significant. No one knows why.

Ockerse also says:[61]

> The high amount of calcium available in the drinking-water in the low-caries areas may however, assist the calcification of the teeth both in utero and after birth up to eight years, making them more caries resistant. The low calcium content in drinking water in the high-caries areas may be responsible for a calcium deficiency during calcification of the teeth, and may be an important contributory causal factor of the high caries-incidence rate.

In any case, as in the case of fluorosis, we may be sure that, while statistical effect on the community may be related to the water supply, effect on any individual is determined by amounts he consumes, *not* by what is in the water.

Basis of the Fluoride-Caries Hypothesis

Since the fluoride-caries hypothesis and the promised reductions in tooth decay are both based on DMF rates, they don't mean anything, and have no scientific importance. They have, and have had, political importance, however, so it is more than idle interest that should make us wonder just how the impossible was accomplished.

We have already seen that high-calcium cities were selected

for the twenty-one cities, but there was far more to the matter than that. In 1948, Dean wrote:[62]

> An inverse variation between endemic dental fluorosis (mottled enamel) and dental caries experience was demonstrated by Dean in 1938. Examination of 236 nine-year-old children of verified continuous residence in the six communities studied, indicated that a higher percentage of caries-free children were found among the users of higher fluoride domestic waters than among the users of lower fluoride domestic waters. This relative freedom from dental caries was present in deciduous as well as permanent teeth, *whether or not the child showed macroscopic evidence of mottled enamel.*

TABLE 2

FLUORIDE VS. INCIDENCE OF CARIES (PERMANENT TEETH)

City	Children Examined	Fluoride in ppm	Percentage Caries-free
Pueblo, Colorado	49	0.6	37
Junction City, Kansas	30	0.7	26
East Moline, Illinois	35	1.5	11
Monmouth, Illinois	29	1.7	55
Galesburg, Illinois	39	1.8	56
Colorado Springs, Colo.	54	2.5	41

The figures in Table 2 are taken from the original article.[63]

It would appear to take some ingenuity and a certain amount of determination to deduce from these data the conclusion Dean drew. But, he did it.

The following year another study, on twelve- to fourteen-year-olds, was done to confirm these "findings." *Although Dean knew that both Galesburg and Monmouth had had major changes in water supply within the lifetime of that group,* they were chosen, for perhaps obvious reasons, to compare with Macomb and Quincy, both also in Illinois.

TABLE 3

DATA FROM THE "GALESBURG-QUINCY STUDY"

	Fluoride in ppm	Calcium in ppm	Carious permanent teeth / 100 children
Galesburg	1.9	62.2	194
Monmouth	1.6	65.0	208
Macomb	0.2	47.1	368
Quincy	0.2	28.2	628

The figures in Table 3 are taken from the original report.[64] On page 884 of the original report, Dean says:

> While on the basis of our present knowledge it appears reasonable to associate the low caries rates observed at Galesburg and Monmouth with the presence of small amounts of fluorides in the domestic water, the possibility that the composition of the water in other respects may also be a factor should not be overlooked.

But neither then, nor since, has he ever mentioned that the "caries-experience rate" seemed to show a much closer relationship to calcium than to fluorine concentration.

CONCLUSIONS FROM THE GALESBURG-QUINCY STUDY

The "caries-experience" figures given above *are* the basis for the statement that there is only from a third to a half as much tooth decay where there are small amounts of fluoride in the water as where there is none. This, in turn, was the basis of the original estimate that reduction from fluoridation would be from 50 to 67 percent.*

When, however, the twenty-one cities were selected to confirm this "hypothesis," Galesburg and Quincy were included, but Monmouth and Macomb were dropped. Also, the study was named the "Galesburg-Quincy Study" which, as you can see

---

* We should note that the "small amount" is 1.8 ppm, *not* 1.0 ppm.

from the figures, permits increasing the reduction to a flat 67 percent, with some to spare.

All later studies have been designed, and their results presented, so as to confirm this "hypothesis" and its figure of 67-percent reduction. It has taken some ingenuity at times, but as we saw in the previous study, they are quite up to it.

When the study of the twenty-one cities was done, the decay rates ranged from 236 at Galesburg to 1037 at Michigan City. These were so grouped and manipulated as to show a "reduction" of about 60 percent.

Since then we have had 60-percent reductions reported from all over the place, including such places as Newburgh and Grand Rapids. Sometimes they are 60 percent of one thing, and sometimes another, but the figure is always the same. Thus they all "confirm" each other.

PROTECTION WITHOUT MOTTLING

The Galesburg-Quincy Study was also used to confirm the statement that protection occurred whether or not there was mottling. This statement was statistical, and *not* based on observation of individuals. It was "confirmed" by the findings at Galesburg, where about half the children had "definite mottling" at age twelve to fourteen, and the other half were not yet so classified. DMF rates in the two groups were said to be about the same, which observation was assumed to have proved that protection was independent of mottling.

THE FLUORIDATION EXPERIMENTS

There is this to be said for Dean and McKay, and to a certain extent for McClure. They published their actual findings in complete and meticulous detail. This was commendable, but it left them very vulnerable. No such mistake has been made at Newburgh or Grand Rapids. No statistician, and no one else outside the group of experimenters, has ever been able to make head or tail of what is behind their published figures. They select and publish figures which come out 60 percent, or will be

60 when the experiments have gone on a little longer. That is as far as you can get.

And actually, it is not worth the effort to try. The figures are based on DMF rates, which, as we have seen, are utterly without meaning. These experiments could not prove anything if they ran a hundred years.

Meanwhile, Blayney, at Evanston, Illinois, was trying to run an honest and scientifically respectable experiment. He refused to be pressured into making premature or unfounded claims. His findings were quite different from the others, and he said so. He was excoriated unmercifully at the Fourth Annual Conference in 1951, for being too honest. Since then we have heard nothing about there even being an experiment at Evanston.

Big Brother Knows Best: Budding Authoritarianism

in Our Public Health Service

IN Chapter 2[1] of this book, I told why fluoridation is unsound medically, and said that sounder alternatives are easily and cheaply available. I presented evidence that the Public Health Service has gone to great lengths to deny the very real danger of chronic fluoride poisoning from the fluoridation of water.

In Chapter 3,[2] I told of mottled enamel and its significance both as a personal blemish and as a manifestation of general toxicosis. I told of the protective action of calcium, and of the danger in adding fluoride artificially to soft waters. And, again, I disclosed the untrustworthy nature of the so-called "scientific case" for fluoridation.

It is an incredible story of chicanery and malfeasance, and because it is incredible, the facts had to speak for themselves. Documentation was not sufficient. Only by quotation *in extenso* could I expect to bring home to the reader that these things had actually been said and done.

Now, having seen *what* has been done, it is time to consider the *how* and the *why*, and what these things mean to the social, political and scientific future of America.

The *how* is quite clear in the record, as we shall see. And where we are going can be deduced from where we are and where we have been. The *why*, on the other hand, is something else again. We may be sure that in any choice of action there is effective motivation, but motives are difficult to prove.

In what we have already discussed, it is hard to tell where stupidity and carelessness leave off and dishonesty begins, and it will be just as hard in the discussion to come. It will also be hard to tell the fortuitous event from the planned, and the schemer from the weak or venal tool.

All this should not blind us to the fact that powerful motives exist, or prevent our considering what they might be. And if we keep possible motives in mind, perhaps the reader can make a pretty good guess where they come in.

POSSIBLE BASIC MOTIVES

As we shall see, there are those both in and out of government who sincerely believe in the *Führer* principle, and who strive to promote totalitarian ways. These are hard to distinguish from the "do-gooders" who promote totalitarianism through good-intentions-gone-crosswise, and without conscious acceptance of totalitarian philosophy. The distinction is not important since the end result is the same.

Then we have the age-old and ever-present empire-building urge of the bureaucrat. The desire for job security, power, and promotion is effective motive for many things, including the unquestioning carrying out of orders, real or imagined.

A government does not operate in a vacuum, however, and its functionaries are often influenced by outside pressures. And when we look, strong potential motives are not hard to find.

First of all is the prospect of direct profit from sale of chemicals and equipment. And you profit twice when a poisonous waste-product, otherwise difficult and expensive to dispose of safely, can be sold.

Even more important, the sale of primary products was at stake. By a vigorous campaign it had been thoroughly established that anyone who said either aluminum utensils or phosphate fertilizer was unsafe was a crack-pot. Soluble aluminum salts are not absorbed from the gut, and they pass through without harm. Also, phosphate was phosphate regardless of its source.

The crack-pots did not know that the fertilizer also contained fluoride, or that the utensils contained fluoride occluded in the aluminum; but the manufacturers did. It was in the course of studies to prove aluminum safe that H. V. Churchill learned that waters which mottled teeth contained fluoride.

It is not known whether the fluoride in aluminum is dangerous, and no one is about to find out. Spira says it is, so he is a crack-pot. I wonder. *The point, however, is not whether it is poisonous. If people even suspected that it might be, it would seriously affect sales.* And the company knew it.

We may also note that the fluoridation promotion embodies apparently irrelevant items. It is said that water is the only important source of fluoride; that plants where fluoride is high contain no more than where it is low; that milk does not contain fluoride regardless of the feed.* [3] All these statements are untrue, and all fit a pattern of motive. But how much better if people could be made to believe that a little fluoride is *good* for you.

A third motive arises from environmental contamination with fluorine. The countryside around aluminum and fertilizer plants is devastated by fluoride fumes to the extent that millions in damages have been paid. But the damage does not stop there, and to prevent the pollution would be so expensive that the millions in damages are considered well spent.

Air and water pollution are also important. The Meuse[4] fog

---

* In this connection, it is interesting that Roholm published pictures of four children with badly disfigured teeth. Their only source of fluorine had been their mothers' milk. The mothers had worked in a cryolite factory and were still liberating enough stored fluorine from their bones to make their milk toxic.

disaster of 1930 was traced to fluoride, and the later Donora and London disasters were probably the same. We are told of the ozone in Los Angeles smog, but not of the hydrofluoric acid. Meanwhile, the fumes settle on the land and are washed down in the rain, and eventually join in the streams with run-off from phosphate-fertilized fields.

In all this, how much better it would be if people could be led to believe that fluoride is beneficial. And in this connection it is interesting to note that when Gerald J. Cox, Ph.D., suggested fluoridation in 1939, and said: "the present trend toward complete removal of fluorine from water and food may need some reversal," he was connected with the Mellon Institute,[5] established by the bequest of the late Andrew Mellon, President of the Aluminum Company of America. The Institute gets most of its income from Alcoa stocks.

No one knows what role these motives have played, but we would fool no one but ourselves if we pretended they do not exist.

How Safe Is "Safe"?

In 1931, three independent reports, by the Smiths,[6] by Velu,[7] and by Churchill,[*8] identified water-borne fluoride as the cause of mottled enamel. In 1932, F. S. McKay, D.D.S., presented to the American Association for the Advancement of Science a paper entitled: "Mottled enamel: A preventable endemic lesion of the teeth that presents a new problem in civic responsibility." In discussing this paper, Churchill said:[9]

> The humble contribution of your speaker was the illumination of the problem of mottled enamel by the demonstrated fact that in all localities studied wherein mottled enamel is

* The actual discovery was by A. W. Petrey, in the Research Laboratories of Aluminum Company of America, New Kensington, Pa., but is credited to his chief, H. V. Churchill, who made the report.

endemic, the water supplies contain more than 2 parts per million of fluorine.[*10]

and farther on, he said:

It would be interesting to compare enamel structure statistically in localities where fluorine is absent from water supply, with enamel from localities where fluorine is present to the normal amount found in American cities (less than 2 ppm). Perhaps it would be revealed that . . . the defect becomes severe enough to be noticed only when the fluorine reaches a critical concentration.

Thus, Churchill *laid down the entire "scientific case" for fluoridation before investigation had even been commenced,* and in spite of the fact that common sense should have told him that fluoride effect would be governed by concentration in the tissues rather than in the water.

"THE MINIMUM THRESHOLD OF TOXICITY"

H. Trendley Dean, D.D.S., was given the job of finding out for the Public Health Service how much fluoride might safely be permitted in a water supply. He quickly learned that the trouble was much more widespread than anyone had supposed, and by 1942 he knew of about 400 cities where fluorosis was endemic.[11]

He also learned that, because of

normal biologic variability, natural differences in sensitivity (or resistance), amount of water drunk, amount of milk consumed, dietary and culinary habits, and doubtless other unrecognizable variables influencing the fluoride intake,[12]

---

[*] Churchill is still quoted as having proved that mottled enamel does not occur where there is less than 2 ppm of fluoride. He actually studied only five places where it was endemic. These had 2.0, 6.0, 11.0, 12.0 and 13.7 ppm, respectively. The place with 2.0 was Colorado Springs, where Dean found 73.8 percent of children to have "definite" mottling. This is hardly proof that none occurs with lesser concentrations.

people using the same water might, or might not, develop mottling; and that wherever there was fluorine in measurable amount, at least some of the people would develop mottling.

It was clear that, if water supplies were to be "safe" for every user, *all* fluoride would have to be removed. It was also clear that there was no feasible way of removing fluoride other than to obtain a new water supply from a fluorine-free source. In many cases this would be impossible and, at best, it would be expensive.

Dean's problem, therefore, ceased to be one of determining what amount of fluoride would be safe for everyone. It became a question of deciding what concentration would cause so much damage to so many people that the city must be required to change its source of water.

Dean set out to establish a maximum tolerance for fluoride by what he likes to call "epidemiological studies." He recognized from the start these had no predictive value regarding the individual. He said:[13]

[This method] is distinctly opposed to the clinical method in which the individual, rather than a population of individuals, is the unit of investigation. In an epidemiological inquiry all observations are related to the group; in a clinical study the observations remain related to the specific individuals under study.

In 1936, he told the American Medical Association:[14]

Although a prognosis with respect to any one individual is obviously unwarranted, it is felt that a prognosis relative to the group response to waters of varying fluoride concentration may be tentatively made at this time.

and that:

The minimal threshold of toxicity in drinking water has not yet been definitely established, but studies to date would suggest that amounts not exceeding one part per million, expressed in terms of fluorine (F), are of no public health significance.*

But before you can decide what is too much damage to too many people, you must first decide how much is too much, and how many is too many. In 1935, Dean wrote:[15]

> For public health purposes we have arbitrarily defined the minimal threshold of fluoride concentration in a domestic water supply as the highest concentration of fluoride incapable of producing a definite degree of mottled enamel in as much as 10 percent of the group examined.

A footnote tells us that "a definite degree of mottled enamel" means mottling which is classified as "very mild" or worse, by his 1935 classification.[16]

As I have proved elsewhere,[17] "questionable" mottling, or mottling so slight as to pass unnoticed, was not and never has been included in the count.

When the above definition of the "minimal threshold" was adopted, Dean believed that not more than 10 percent of children would develop "definite mottling" from water containing 1 part per million of fluorine. By 1938, however, he had learned that the damage would be much higher. He wrote[18] that where the fluoride content was just over 1.0 part per million, the examiner might find "very mild" or "mild" fluorosis in 25 to 30 percent of children. He also stated that even where there was less fluoride "sporadic cases of very mild degree are occasionally observed."

There were two things Dean could do. He could lower his "minimal threshold" till only 10 percent were damaged or he could raise the figure for permissible damage. He chose to do the latter. However, at the same time he adopted a new method of reporting in which the percent of damage did not appear.

---

* This statement will be discussed further, under "weasel words."

He invented what he calls the "community index of dental fluorosis." [19]

On the basis of Dean's work, the U. S. Treasury Department (which then had jurisdiction in such matters) set 1.0 part per million as the maximum tolerance for fluorine in community water supplies.[20] As we have seen, this was expected to produce from 25 to 30 percent of definite mottling. We should also note that *other toxic effects of fluorine were not even considered.*

Putting Fluoride In vs. Taking It Out

That was in 1942, and the Public Health Service did not endorse the addition of fluoride to water supplies till 1951.

You might reasonably expect to find a definite difference between the amount of damage you *must* use tax money to *prevent* and the amount you *may* use tax money to *produce.* Apparently there is a difference, but not of the sort you would expect. In 1946, the Public Health Service *raised* the tolerance for fluorine in water supplies from 1.0 part per million to 1.5 parts per million. This was *not* done because of any new proofs of safety, but simply because 1.2 parts per million was already being used in the so-called experiment in artificial fluoridation at Newburgh, N. Y., and they had to make it legal.

In 1952, Bruce Forsyth, D.D.S., Assistant Surgeon General of the Public Health Service, said in testimony before the Delaney Committee:[21]

> You see actually the safe amount had been set even before fluoridation, at 1½ parts per million in our Public Health water standards. So we don't recommend more than 1 to 1½ parts of fluorine per million parts of water.

And F. J. Maier, B.S., Senior Sanitary Engineer of the Public Health Service, was not talking about taking fluoride out but putting it in when, in 1951, he told the 4th Annual Conference of State Dental Directors that:[22]

> The criterion we have been using is that if there is some 10 to 20 percent fluorosis in the community, that would not be objectionable,* because in those places the degree of intensity is not greater than the accepted definition of 'mild.'†[23]

It is interesting, but perhaps not surprising, that there was no word of protest from the dental directors, and they spent the next two days deciding how they would "put over" fluoridation.

THE WEASEL WORDS

It is doubtful if many people other than public health employees would countenance the addition of fluoride to water supplies if they knew that it was expected to injure even a single child. It has been necessary to convince people that fluoridation is, in fact, completely safe.

In doing this, the primary tools have been equivocation and prevarication. Outright lies are rarely used except when so tightly cornered under cross-examination that there is no other way out.

The Public Health Service has adopted special definitions for certain words and phrases, which permit its representatives to appear to be saying one thing when they actually mean something very different. You find awkward turns of phrase, and apparently superfluous words, thrown in for no apparent reason. When you do, it is a fairly safe bet that the statement does not mean what it appears to say.

* This use of the word "objectionable" will be discussed in the next section, "The Weasel Words."

† As we have seen, "the accepted definition of mild" includes gross disfigurement. Even so, the statement is not true. One PHS study reported two places with "moderate" and one with "severe" mottling. Yet in neither place was the concentration of fluoride as much as 1 ppm, or the incidence of mottling as high as 20 percent. There are other similar reports.

For example, Thomas Parran, M.D., who was Surgeon General during Dean's early work, recently wrote an article referring repeatedly to the "safety" of fluoridation. In it he says:[24]

> . . . scientific evidence indicates overwhelmingly the safety to the population.

He will, of course, be quoted as saying fluoridation is "safe," but if he is challenged he can say: "I did not say it was safe for any individual. I merely said it was safe for the population." As we have seen, that merely means that he does not expect more than about 20 percent of people to be injured.

We have already encountered the term "minimal threshold of toxicity," which to most people would mean something like Churchill's "critical concentration" below which no effect could be detected. By judicious use of this term, instead of the proper term "maximum tolerance" it has been possible to mislead any number of good people.

We have also seen that *by definition,* fluorosis produced by water containing 1 part per million of fluorine is "not objectionable," and "has no public health significance." At several points, these private meanings were all that stood between the Public Health Service representatives and perjury before the Delaney Committee. And, when John W. Knutson, D.D.S., said:[25]

> . . . if we get one objectionable case of mottled enamel in a community, even if it involved the examination of a thousand children, that would be too much fluoride.

he was perfectly safe, because, by definition 1 part per million of fluoride cannot produce "an objectionable case."

By definition, fluorosis is "endemic" only if produced where there is more than 1 part per million of fluorine. Any produced by lesser amounts is a "sporadic case." Then, when we privately define "mottled enamel" as "chronic *endemic* dental fluorosis," we can say, quite truthfully, that mottled enamel is never produced by water containing less than one part per million of fluoride.

There are more, but these should be enough to illustrate the process. When one of your carefully worded equivocations is misquoted, you can quote the misquotation and the onus of the falsehood is on the person you quote. What could be lovelier? The fluoridation literature is no safe place for the careless reader, and you dare take nothing, not even a single word, for granted. And you *must* be aware of the private definitions.

The Totalitarian Concept of Public Health

As we have seen, the Public Health Service proposes that a proportion of people be actively harmed in order that they, or others, may be "benefited." The intent is: 21-47 percent to get "questionable" or "definite" mottling and the associated toxicosis; and 20 percent to be "protected," till age 14, from caries.* [26] The excuse that they expect the damage to be trivial will not wash, at least insofar as the leaders are concerned. Their attempts to discount and conceal the probability of harm were not made in absent-minded moments. They had to be planned policy.

Dean, moreover, must have known and shared the sentiments of Francis Heyroth, M.D., Assistant Director of the Kettering Institute, who served with him on the nine-man Ad Hoc Committee that approved fluoridation for the National Research Council. Heyroth wrote:[27]

> The question of the effect of water containing 1 p.p.m. upon patients with severe impairment of kidney function

* Their "case" is based on the 21 cities so, for this purpose, we can accept those figures at face value. In 5 cities with 0.9-1.3 ppm fluorine, 78.0% of children had decay. 21.5% had definite mottling and an additional 32.2% had questionable mottling. In 7 cities with 0.0-0.1 ppm, the corresponding figures were 97.6%, 0.6%, and 6.5% respectively. Subtracting we get: 19.6% less children had decay, 20.9% more had definite mottling, and 25.7% more had questionable mottling. 20.9 + 25.7 = 46.6.

requires special consideration in view of the fact that radiologic evidence of chronic fluorosis has been found in two persons with severe kidney disease who died at the early ages of 22 and 23 years, respectively . . .

In any event, *the risk that such patients might be harmed by the fluoridation of water appears to be small in comparison with the dental benefits to be obtained.* (Italics mine.)

We are told that this is a "calculated risk" comparable with what each of us takes whenever he crosses a street. The difference is obvious.

Each of us decides for himself to cross or not to cross, and whether the advantage to be gained by crossing warrants the risk. Fluoridation has more in common with the calculation of risk by a general who decides how many men he is willing to lose when he sends shock-troops into battle.

THE GREATEST GOOD FOR THE GREATEST NUMBER

Except as pertaining to troops, the idea that government may sacrifice individuals to the public good is something new in American political philosophy. The idea of the greatest good to the greatest number is naïvely accepted in college classrooms, with no thought to who decides what is good and how he brings it to pass.

The obvious answer is that it is decided by "experts" who compel others to behave accordingly. When you recognize this the idea is not so appealing—unless you expect to be one of the experts. And being a minor expert is not enough. You must be top dog or eventually you, too, will get it.

"BROADER HORIZONS" FOR PUBLIC HEALTH

America was founded on the concept that all men have equal rights in the eyes of God and the Law. The Constitution was designed to protect us in the enjoyment of our rights. They may not be infringed except with due process of law, and then only insofar as their exercise endangers the rights of others.

One of these rights is the right to decide, each for himself, what shall be done to his own body. Accordingly, health departments have had "police power" to *protect* us from conditions and practices which might endanger our health. The idea that they may also *promote* our health by doing things to us without our consent, is new and different.

I have discussed elsewhere[28] the implications of the new-found "conviction" of the Public Health Service "that physical fitness, for civilians as well as for troops, was a duty owed the Nation"[29]—a duty to be enforced, willy-nilly and regardless of consequences, by the Public Health Service and its emissaries.

Recently a state health officer, dependent as they all are on the Public Health Service for funds and guidance, suggested that he be given power of emergency commitment, for mental disease, under the quarantine laws and without due process of law. He said: "Under the law all matters of the health and welfare of the people of the State come under the State Department of Health.[30]

And the Public Health Service, itself, has said:

> We have begun to think of the patient as a total person. We are concerned today not only with his medical problems . . . but also with his personal problems, his reactions and his feelings.
>
> Modern medicine knows that unless we deal with the total man we do not meet the problems of his illness. The . . . health department is . . . attempting to marshal the forces which can help him as a person.

To be sure, the article dealt with tuberculosis, a communicable disease. But in the same issue was an editorial by an Assistant Surgeon General.[31] This was entitled "An Opportunity for Leadership," and urged that the ideas and methods in the article I have quoted "serve as a guide mark to other and newer public health activities . . . in an era when chronic diseases and the problems of the aging are beginning to draw increasing attention."

COMPULSORY MEDICATION

In this grandiose new concept of public health, there is only one major obstacle. We shrink from compulsory medication even in communicable disease, while for noncontagious disease it has been considered unthinkable. That is where fluoridation comes in. It is to serve as the first legal precedent for compulsory medication in noncommunicable disease. That is its sole purpose, and so far it has done all right.

In 1950, F. J. Maier, of the Public Health Service, said:[32]

> Conversely, the discovery of the role of optimum amounts of fluorides in water has led to the concept that the treatment of drinking water might include the addition of specific substances to prevent disease.

This, of course, is no longer treatment of *water,* but treatment of *people.* And when you get through using your water supply as vehicle for miscellaneous medicines, what do you use for water, or as vehicle for other drugs?

In the case of *Kaul* vs. *City of Chehalis,* Justice Donworth said:[33]

> By [fluoridating the water] the municipal authorities . . . arrogate to themselves the sole right to decide what medicine is good for the health of the water consumers, and thereby the municipal water system becomes a direct conduit for the transportation of medicine* [34] from the apothe-

---

* The much-parroted PHS quibble, that fluoridation is not medication because it treats no disease, is beneath contempt. Call it what you will, the fluoride is used to act on people's bodies without their consent. Moreover, while we speak loosely of treating disease, we don't actually treat diseases. We treat people for, or to prevent, disease. In the Kaul case, Justice Hill said: "If, however, it is the position of respondent city and its experts that, while giving a preventive prescription is practicing medicine, the prescription, when filled, is not medicine and, when used, is not medication, they are dealing in refinements which escape the lay mind and which are not reflected in current terminology."

cary's pestle to the patient without the latter's consent. Thus will the people be deprived of a very important part of their constitutional liberty under our republican form of government and the police state will be substituted for the police power of the state.

and Justice Hamley said:[35]

What future proposals may be made to treat noncontagious diseases by adding ingredients to our water supply, or food, or air, only time will tell. When that day arrives, those who treasure their personal liberty will look in vain for a constitutional safeguard. The answer will be: "You gave the constitution away in the Kaul case."

ALL OR NONE

Once you accept any part of totalitarian philosophy, there are no halfway points. Either each person has the right to decide for himself what shall be done to him—to make his own mistakes and take the consequences—or the government has a duty to do things to him "for his own good" or for that of society. We have seen the consequences of the latter view carried to their logical conclusions in Italy, Germany, and Russia.

But they are also becoming apparent in this country, and we don't have to look too hard to find them.

We have noted the ruthless willingness of the Public Health Service to sacrifice up to 20 percent of the people to just one of its projects. We are aware that whole populations have been used as subjects for the fluoridation "experiments" without their consent. The Public Health Service has used people as subjects for other experiments under conditions of duress wherein free consent was impossible.[36] We hanged Germans for this same offense.

We have recently seen persons incarcerated, without process of law, for "political insanity." Perhaps we were reminded of the intensive drive by the Public Health Service to invade the field of "mental health," and remember, unpleasantly, what happened to "undesirable persons" in Germany as a result of the same development.

THE TYRANNY OF THE MAJORITY

George F. Lull, M.D., Secretary of the American Medical Association, recently came out flat-footed for the totalitarian way. He said:[37]

> With all due allowance for the democratic process, it must be held that the resistance to fluoridation of water supplies is a minority opinion and that the majority must rule.

The plain fact is that if the majority had been allowed to rule, there would be no fluoridation. In most places where it has been left to the people it has been rejected, and usually by overwhelming majorities. *But that is not the point.*

Someone should tell the good doctor that our Constitution provides, and the American Medical Association has always held, that in matters of personal health the opinion of the majority is without force and the *individual* must decide.

Madison once said:[38]

> Wherever the real power in a government lies, there is the danger of oppression. In our government the real power lies in the majority of the community, and the invasion of private rights is chiefly to be apprehended, not from acts of government contrary to the sense of its constituents but from acts in which the government is the mere instrument of the major number of the constituents.

and the Supreme Court of the United States has held:[39]

> It must be conceded that there are such [private] rights in every free government beyond the control of the State. A government which recognized no such rights, which held the lives, the liberty and the property of its citizens, subject at all times to the absolute disposition and unlimited

control of even the most democratic depository of power, is after all but a despotism. It is true it is a despotism of the many, of the majority, if you choose to call it so, but it is none the less a despotism. It may well be doubted if a man is to hold all that he is accustomed to call his own . . . under the unlimited dominion of others, whether it is not wiser that this power should be exercised by one man than by many.

It is fortunate that majority opinion *has* rejected, and largely prevented, fluoridation of water supplies. The fact remains that rejecting it by majority vote is as wrong as accepting it by majority vote. *Even the contemplation of fluoridation has no place in a democracy. It lies wholly outside the proper sphere of governmental action.*

Public Health Law and Authoritarian Science

Our public health law stems from a basic dilemma. The law must, insofar as possible, be based on sound scientific knowledge. Yet science, frozen into law, ceases to be science. Law, on the other hand, cannot remain law and still bow to the necessary instability of free scientific opinion.

The solution has been to create a special legislature called a *board* of health, composed of men capable of responding to the climate of professional opinion much as the regular legislature responds to the climate of political opinion. This board is given broad powers to write such rules and regulations as it deems necessary for *protection* of the *public* health. These have the force of law.

Health *departments* are then given such police power as is necessary for administration and enforcement of the rules and regulations of the board. Thus, the legislative and administrative functions are properly separated, and the judicial function is fulfilled by our ordinary courts of law.

All this spells nothing but trouble for health departments bent on expanding their powers, and "promoting" the welfare of the individual citizen. For this they need a free hand, and autocratic power. One way to these is by controlling or by-passing the boards. Perhaps they can even be abolished or rendered impotent. Meanwhile, however, much can be accomplished by controlling the "climate of professional opinion."

SCIENCE BY EDICT

It is generally considered that science was born when Galileo dropped balls of different weight from the Tower of Pisa and, by proving that they fell at the same rate, also proved that facts take precedence over the dicta of authority.

In science there can be neither orthodoxy nor heresy. The science of today is superstition tomorrow, and only facts have permanence. No one is a scientist who clings to any opinion, however widely shared, if it conflicts in the slightest degree with any fact known to him.

We recognize the impending doom of science in Russia, when scientists are required to accept Lysenko's theories of heredity. Whether the theories are true or false is irrelevant. The point is that acceptance is mandatory. "Truth" is established by edict, not by free exchange in the market-place of ideas.

We look down our noses at the benighted Russians, and never think how far down the same road we have come.

POLIO AND TOOTH DECAY

We forget that, on a certain morning at 10 o'clock, Salk vaccine became, by edict, a safe and effective means for partial prevention of polio. This set off a planned spontaneous demonstration and a game of follow-my-leader that even the Russians could hardly surpass.

Perhaps we didn't notice how exactly this followed the pattern set by fluoridation which, on April 24, 1951, was pronounced by the Surgeon General to be a safe and effective means for partial prevention of tooth decay.

No one knows what would have happened if the vaccine had been safe. It wasn't, and we were forceably reminded that there was something wrong with the method by which we had been assured of its safety. The method would have been just as wrong if the vaccine *had* been safe, and the greatest thing since soap.

The American Medical Association was quick to recognize what was wrong, and said:[40]

> Whereas, There are traditional methods by which investigators and scientists in all fields announce and critically review discoveries and applications thereof: be it
>
> *Resolved,* That we reaffirm our confidence in the established methods of announcing new and possibly beneficial methods in the treatment and prevention of disease; and be it further
>
> *Resolved,* that we reaffirm the need for presentation of reports on medical research before established scientific groups, allowing free discussion and criticism, and the publication of such reports, including methods employed and data acquired on which the results and conclusions are based, in recognized scientific publications.

Yet this same American Medical Association espoused the authoritarian way when its House of Delegates "endorsed the principle" of fluoridation,* and when it permitted itself, without protest, to be represented as one of the prime sponsors.

This was done despite the fact that the "traditional methods," as above outlined, were never followed. It was done in face of the further fact that the "principle" contemplates compulsory medication, whereas even in the case of polio, a contagious disease, it was to be, to a degree and for the present, voluntary.

It is true that the Secretary of American Medical Association twice told the Congress that "the House of Delegates did not urge or recommend that any communities undertake to fluoridate their water supplies." The fact remains that no attempt has been made to make this clear either to the public or to physicians.

The Secretary has even told the public:[37]

* At Los Angeles, 1951.

. . . the unscrupulous opponents of fluoridation have spread the impression that the American Medical Association did not endorse this public health measure. The fact is that it did, and that it stands by its endorsement. . . . Both the A.M.A. Council on Pharmacy and Chemistry and the A.M.A. Council on Foods and Nutrition expressed themselves definitely to the effect that fluoridation is safe. If this is not an endorsement—what is it?

If he really wants to know, it is clearly "science by edict." And also, if he wants to know, it is beyond the powers of either the Councils or the House of Delegates to promulgate such edicts. If the American Medical Association had a supreme court the "endorsements" would undoubtedly be declared unconstitutional, and of no effect.

Concoction and Appropriation of Authority

In science, and in the professions, there is no such thing as an authority. The essence of authority is the ability to *command* unquestioning obedience or belief. The essence of expertness, on the other hand, is merely the possession of unusual knowledge or skill in a particular field.

At the same time, the expert may be so respected that he is *accorded* an unquestioning belief he cannot command, while the one in authority may rely solely on voluntary belief or obedience. Where these things are true, the distinction between expert and authority may not be obvious. This can be useful.

A FIELD WITH NO COMPETING EXPERTS

In building up an expert whose word will go unchallenged, it helps to select a field where there are no established experts. Fluoridation was ideal for the purpose. It was outside the scope of medicine because it dealt with teeth. It was not dentistry because it was preventive medicine. It was not public health because tooth decay is noncontagious. It was outside water-works practice because it treated people rather than water. It was an uninhabited no-man's land, yet close enough to each of these other fields to command interested but uncritical attention.

Dean's basic studies were never published in any professional publication. The fifteen reports which give his methods and data were all published in Public Health Reports. This is a wholly controlled "house organ" of the Public Health Service. There is no editorial selection, and no opportunity for contrary evidence or debate. Even its readership was largely limited to public-health personnel. Most of the personnel, like everyone else for that matter, knew little and cared less about tooth decay or fluorine or both.

Paralleling these, he published thirteen other articles in the same period, some here, some there, in American and foreign periodicals and telling *about* his work.[41] He also made personal appearances before interested groups, including the American Medical Association, American Dental Association, American Public Health Association, and American Association for the Advancement of Science.

At the same time he became active and influential in the American Dental Association and the American Association for the Advancement of Science. He wrote the report on mottled enamel for the American Dental Association[42] and engineered the symposium for the American Association for the Advancement of Science in 1941,[43] and again in 1946.[44]

Then he became active in the American Water Works Association, American Public Health Association, National Research Council, International Association for Dental Research (publishers of the highly respected *Journal of Dental Research*), and the American Association of Dental Editors. In each he was the only source of information on fluorine as related to teeth, and he did yeoman service in promoting himself and the cause of fluoridation.

Each step made the next one easier, and he ended up with countless appointments and assignments, honors, and medals, wrote chapters for textbooks and symposia, and published seventeen more articles about fluoridation, made uncounted personal appearances, and was all the time on the payroll of the Public Health Service.

Dean became the universally recognized high priest of fluoridation, but first came the build-up.

THE CLAQUE AND THE CHANT

The best way to become recognized as an expert is to write articles which are quoted. Dean and McClure started this by quoting themselves and each other. Soon they were quoted by others, and they could quote, in support of their conclusions, others who were merely parroting them. This helped.

It also helped when other Public Health Service personnel started to chant that Dean had proved "conclusively" that fluoridation was safe, that the resulting fluorosis was unobjectionable, and that it would reduce tooth decay by about two thirds.

It was a catchy tune, and soon everyone was singing. Those who didn't know all the words improvised some and sang along with the rest. Why should that spoil their fun?

THE TRANSFER OF AUTHORITY

In 1948, Dean was made Director of the National Institute of Dental Research (of the Public Health Service). By this move, his prestige was extended, first to the work of other personnel, and then to the Institute. He began to talk about what "we" have proved by "our" research.

The next easy step was for the Surgeon General to speak with authority on the subject of fluoridation, and urge its adoption. Then came the edict.

The Usurpation of Power

The Constitution did not contemplate the exercise of police power by the federal government within the states except in regulating interstate commerce, and on Government property, bought with the consent of the legislatures for the erection of needful federal buildings. Neither did it give power to "promote the progress of science and useful arts" except "by securing for limited times to authors and inventors the exclusive right to their respective writings and discoveries."

When Congressman Wier, of Minnesota, introduced in the 83rd Congress, H. R. 2341, a Bill to protect the public health from the dangers of fluorination of water, the cry was raised that this was improper interference by Congress in matters which should be decided locally. State health departments might properly make regulations as to how fluoridation should be carried out, but neither they nor the Congress might tell any community that it must or must not fluoridate.

And who should raise this cry but the Public Health Service and its toadies! Yet in the testimony, John W. Knutson, Assistant Surgeon General and Chief Dental Officer of the Public Health Service, said:[45]

> The responsibilities of the Public Health Service were clear: to make the facts about fluoridation known to State and local health agencies, and to provide them with technical assistance. . . . We could do no less and still meet our obligations as a national health agency.

The "technical assistance" included such things as a propaganda movie for drumming up sentiment for fluoridation in local communities.[46] And one government witness was overheard to say: "This local autonomy business is the best gimmick we have. It lets us go right to the city councils, and prevents interference by Congress or the boards of health." He might well have added: "or the Constitution."

CONTROL BY SUBSIDY

Health departments have never been noted for biting the hand that feeds them. And, unlike some dogs who stay home and starve with their masters, they will cower to anyone from whom they expect a hand-out.

Boards of health have made the rules, but for a time could supply no funds for their administration. Health departments obtained from the legislatures such appropriations as they could make seem reasonable, and had to scrounge for anything beyond that.

But when the Public Health Service was given billions to dole out in subsidies, all this was changed.

Health officers were offered such money and power as they had never dreamed possible. All they had to do was follow "suggestions" and it was theirs. Legislatures and boards of health could go fly a kite, or, better yet, also do what the Public Health Service wanted. And the primary evil lay in the subsidies, not the giving of orders. The U. S. Supreme Court has unanimously held: "It is hardly lack of due process for the Government to regulate that which it subsidizes." [47]

It was definitely "orders from the boss" when the Surgeon General told the State and Territorial Health Officers, in 1953, that, as public health workers,[48] they were[49]

> . . . called upon to exercise a high degree of public health statesmanship. The skeptics must be convinced that our epidemiological and laboratory studies are valid and that the benefits of fluoridation are not to be discarded lightly in the face of uninformed opposition.

He was considerate enough not to remind them that they were less informed than the skeptics. Neither did he propose that they inform themselves. They were to go out and promote. This, of course, they were already doing, but they must do better.

Public Health Statesmanship

In Russia, an edict that Lysenko's theories are true must be accepted. It is backed by threat of liquidation, and there is no need for "skeptics to be convinced" that the "studies are valid."

An edict that Dean's theories are true is not so simple. Dissenters have been attacked personally, their subsidies have been withdrawn or their appointments cancelled, but there are always some who cannot be bought or intimidated.

In the final analysis, it must be made to appear that the edict, like the rules and regulations of the boards of health, merely reflects the "climate of professional opinion." *But, in the case of fluoridation,* the plain fact is that *there is no climate of professional opinion.*

Most physicians and dentists will tell you quite frankly that they know nothing about fluoridation except what they have been told, chiefly through the same channels from which laymen have gotten their information. They have made no attempt to examine the evidence, and have either accepted unsupported statements at face value, or have refused to do so.

The Public Health Service knows this, and wisely warns against paying any attention to the opinions of individual physicians or dentists. In 1954, Knutson was asked by Congressman Warburton:[50]

> W. Then in the case of a dentist who . . . asks me to support the public health position . . . am I to assume that he knows or does not know what he is talking about from his own practical experience?
> K. I would not advise you to assume it, sir . . . [until] the validity of the claim . . . has been tested and reconfirmed by competent investigators.

"Competent investigators" are, of course, those who can be *depended* upon to support the official viewpoint. One takes no chances on others, even when they concur, and the reason is clear. At the 4th Annual Conference, the State Dental Directors were told:[51]

> The unfortunate thing is that some of the research work-ers are going around the country telling the public they cannot recommend fluoridation. That is going to happen in your community. It is happening all over the United States, so you are going to have to combat it.

THE COMPETENT INVESTIGATORS

Blayney, of Evanston, and others who testified against fluorida-tion before the Delaney Committee are obviously not competent investigators, and have, by one means or another, been more or less effectively silenced.

The *competent* investigators, of course, all parrot and lend their prestige to the party line in its entirety. This, in itself, speaks volumes as to their credibility. Nevertheless, it seems worthwhile to take a quick look at a few of them individually.

We will ignore, for the moment, the public health employees and Armstrong of Minnesota, whom we discussed in Chapter 2.

Cox, who first suggested fluoridation, tells us, among other inter-esting things, that "the incidence of stiff backs in this country is nil." He says: "We know the effects on bones and teeth . . . are the results of the actual amount of fluoride ingested, rather than merely the concentration in the water." However, he goes on to say that "engineers and chemists can guarantee that the fluorine content of the water supply falls below the level which can cause any of the recognized injuries," and may even pro-vide "a statistically constant intake of fluorine by seasonal vari-ation of the dosage." He concludes:[52]

> A very important fact remains to be established, one now guessed through certain faulty assumptions: What is the optimum amount of fluorine, and I mean the true optimum, not an arbitrary one, for conferring caries resistant teeth to children of various ages?

The very existence of an "optimum amount" is faulty assumption. It will differ with each individual, and his own writings prove that he knows it.

R. F. Soggnaes, D.D.S., is Dean of the Harvard School of Dental Medicine. In 1937-38, he spent three months on the remote island of Tristan da Cunha to learn why the natives had almost no tooth decay. He now tells us that the water contained 0.2 part per million of fluorine, but that the "average diet" provided an additional 1.5 milligrams per day from fish. (This is the equivalent of an extra 1.6 quarts of water with 1.0 part per million of fluorine.)

He now tells us that:[53]

> . . . the islanders were found to have a threshold degree of mottled enamel and a fluoride content of the teeth close to the amount reported in United States communities with 1 ppm F in the drinking water.

He lets us assume from the fact that he advocates fluoridation that what he found there was not objectionable. He never mentions any more that 60 percent of the upper central incisors of children between six and twenty showed white spots; or that these "were well demarcated from the unaffected portions of the tooth surfaces," or that the "lesions were obvious enough to be revealed at the first smile of many of the younger inhabitants." [54]

Neither does he tell us that deciduous as well as permanent teeth were affected. He lets himself be quoted as saying the people lived exclusively on fish, whereas no one can live on 300 grams of fish per day, and he knows the diet consisted of eggs, milk, meat, potatoes, and vegetables, supplemented by fish.

Then we have Harold Hodge, Ph.D., who supplements pseudo-science with pseudomathematics, and uses the wrong weasel words even after Dean has told him they are wrong.[55]

He tells us[56] that:

> The mathematical relationship between the severity of mottling and the level of fluoride in the drinking water gives

an exceptional reliability to this prediction . . . that the margin of safety for mild mottling is two-fold;

and goes on to say that:

> The principal interest in the statistical nature of mottling lies in the hitherto unconsidered question as to what is responsible for the more severe response in a few children . . . at present we have no indication of what factors control the severity of mottling.

I could cite any number more, but these are fair samples of the fact that the "competent investigators," without exception, *disregard facts known to them,* when they subscribe to the "fluorine-dental caries hypothesis" and "proofs of safety"; and, as we said before, anyone who does this is not a scientist.

THE PLAGIARISTS AND THE HAND-OUTS

> *"In one word, [Nicholai Ivanovitch Lobechevski] gave me the secret of success in mathematics. 'Plagiarize. . . . Only be sure always to call it, please, research.'"*
>
> *Ballad by Tom Lehrer*

The advantages of plagiarism to the plagiarizer are well known, but we tend to forget that there may also be advantages in having your work plagiarized.

A recent article on the safety of fluoridation by a public health employee says:[57]

> Several reviews have been published lately, and there is little point in going over the same ground in detail. Hence this paper will be essentially a review of reviews.

Needless to say, the factual content was meagre and unreliable, but it was one more item of incessant repetition, by which "a colossal lie, if repeated often enough, will be accepted as truer than truth." Now, it is characteristic of rumor that it

changes, wildly, with each repetition and soon bears no resemblance to the original report. These repetitions, on the other
hand, resemble each other so exactly, both in style and word-
ing, that one suspects they were mostly written with the same
pen.

It is an easy way to a fast buck to submit a government hand-
out for publication under your own name. This is common
practice in the lay press and, apparently, also in the "scientific"
press, where it saves one the trouble of doing one's own plagiariz-
ing.

THE ST. LOUIS "STUDY"

One of the references cited in the article I just quoted was
the one by Knutson which I discussed in Chapter 2, and needs
no further comment. Another was the highly-touted "study"
by a committee of the St. Louis Medical Society.[58] This I mentioned, but it needs further notice.

In a bibliography of 67 references, there are three articles by
Dean. Not one of these was a report of his studies. They were
articles, written later, *about* his studies.

The study quotes such "authorities" as Herman Hilleboe,
M.D., State Health Commissioner of New York, saying:

> These results [in Newburgh and Kingston] bear out studies
> made in other areas of the country, where persons have
> been drinking naturally fluoridated water all their lives with
> utmost safety.

and Winston Tucker, M.D., Health Commissioner of Evanston,
Illinois, saying:

> I am not aware of any evidence published in the medical
> literature showing that there is an increase of any disease
> which could be attributed to fluorine in concentration of
> one part per million in a public water supply.

It accuses Congressman A. L. Miller (former State Health
Officer of Nebraska, and a convert *against* fluoridation after

being responsible for its adoption in Washington, D. C.) of having "tortured the meaning of words" and having

> fallen into serious factual error in using inappropriate vital statistics in evaluating the incidence of circulatory disease as a cause of death in Grand Rapids, on which point he has been most clearly and courteously set straight by W. B. Prothro, M.D., Public Health Director of Grand Rapids.

Possibly the congressman did use inappropriate statistics, but apparently so did Prothro. He just applied for, and received, a grant of $5000 from the Public Health Service to find out why deaths from heart disease, cancer, "stroke," diabetes, and arteriosclerosis are so much higher in Grand Rapids than elsewhere in the state.

Consequently, we cannot take it very seriously when C. V. Tossy, M.D., of the Michigan Department of Health, is quoted as saying:

> Vital statistics in Grand Rapids have been studied in comparison with the rest of the state, and there are no differences that could be attributed to fluoridation of the water. There have been no adverse effects of any kind noted.

In short, the St. Louis study boils down to rumor and unsubstantiated opinion, rather than scientific evaluation—plus, as I mentioned before, some quite appalling nonsense.

BEHAVIOR-CENTERED HEALTH EDUCATION

We hear much in public-health circles, these days, about something called "behavior-centered health education." What this means was well stated to me by a former teacher of mine, who said:

> We are under no obligation to tell people the truth. They wouldn't understand it anyway. Our duty is to tell them whatever is necessary to make them do what they ought to do.

It was also well stated by Frank Bull, D.D.S., Director of Dental Health for Wisconsin, when he said:[59]

> When . . . we have decided that fluoridation or any other procedure is a public health measure then we must tell the public that they should adopt that program and explain to them how and why we arrived at these conclusions without creating unnecessary doubt or suspicion in their minds.

THE FOURTH ANNUAL CONFERENCE

In June of 1951, the State Dental Directors were called to Washington to "confer" with the Public Health Service and the Children's Bureau, and this same Frank Bull was given the task of telling them how to put over fluoridation in their respective states.

The proceedings of this conference, which we have referred to before, is an incredible document which must be seen to be believed. After initial release it was strictly "classified" [60] and even congressmen have been unable to obtain it.

The conferees were told that if they wanted to do something that was not within the definition of public health, "they have to embroider the definition a little bit and make it a little more complicated, and then it's justified."

Bull told them how to "build a fire under" the local medical and dental societies, how to rig endorsements, how to draw in the press, how to use civic organizations ("the PTA is a honey"), how to give the business to chemists and engineers (he referred to them as astrologers) and how to play off one group against another. They were to ridicule all opposition and, if possible, to prevent its being heard, and *never,* if it could possibly be avoided, let the matter come to a vote of the people.

He told them what to say and what not to say, and what words to avoid. They must anticipate and have some sort of answer to every possible objection.

They were advised to admit that fluoridation would cause fluorosis, but to say that fluorosis in that amount made teeth more beautiful. "You have got to have an answer. Maybe you have a better one." And he told them to avoid any mention or discussion of toxicity because "I don't know any answer to that one."

In the whole three days, there was no word of protest, and the Directors came home to put in practice what they had been taught. I leave you to judge how well they learned their lesson.

At this same conference, Bull said:[61]

> How can you expect the dentists of your state to go very far on fluoridation when they have never heard anything on it? . . . You have to keep this thing before them . . . on the state meeting level. And when you have it on that level, don't get someone on the program who ends up with, "But I don't think you should do it." . . . Are we trying to promote this thing, or do we want to argue about it? . . .
>
> Your local component dental societies also have got to have programs on fluoridation. Who can supply them? The committee from the state society and your state board of health can. When they have the first meeting at the local level, that is the time to get the press in, and as a rule we don't even wait for that.

That is how the dentists who had "never heard anything on fluoridation" were given the word. They were also told that if they opposed it they would be accused of feathering their nests by trying to promote tooth decay, and that:[62]

> In this matter of fluoridation it is not sufficient for a practicing dentist to "damn with faint praise" when a patient wishes to discuss the process. He should not pass on to the patient his personal opinions . . . but should use the facts which are readily available to him.

THE AMERICAN DENTAL ASSOCIATION

It should be clear that the intensity with which the American Dental Association is promoting fluoridation does not spring from grass-roots pressure. We know the "endorsement" was engineered, at headquarters, by Dean. Other organizations have also "endorsed," however, and none have been such zealous promoters on that account.

A partial explanation may be found in the fact that, "way back when," the entire "research fund" collected by the American Dental Association from its members was turned over to the Public Health Service to use. The danger in this was pointed out by Tainter,[63] in 1943, but the damage was already done. Those who had thus used the funds must justify their act by proving that they had been well spent. The result *had* to be good, and the result was fluoridation.

The Enthusiasts

It would be wrong, in closing, not to mention certain outstanding performers whose free-wheeling imaginations and lack of restraint make the more cautious experts seem almost respectable.

Many of these are in our health departments, and we have already noted the one who says that if there is any calcium deficiency people will have no bones or teeth.

Then there was the anonymous spokesman for the California State Department of Health who said: "Neither can the content be changed by boiling or freezing the water";[64] and the minor genius in the Illinois Department of Health who wrote an inquirer that if she boiled away half of the water from a container of water with 1 part per million of fluorine, what was left would contain only one-half part per million.[65]

Then we have Professor Leicester, of San Francisco, who says that whoever made that last statement was an absolute fool. However, a few minutes later he says: "These questions about what happens if you take soups that are a little bit more concentrated . . . have no bearing on the matter."[66]

He claims to be a biochemist, but says that the concentration of fluoride in the blood reflects the concentration in the water, so that, below 1 part per million, fluoride leaves the bones instead of entering.

He says that all people drink the same amount of water, and any differences are due only to climate, and that there is no scientific evidence to the contrary. He even says that scientific experiments are being conducted to prove this is true.[67]

He says that a fluoride ion is a fluoride ion wherever it comes from and its actions in the body are identical in every respect, and in the same meeting says:[68]

> The fluoride in smog is chiefly hydrofluoric acid. It is also in the air in various concentrations . . . and deposited on all the foliage around, which cattle eat and have been poisoned by it . . .
>
> The fluoride that is added to the drinking water . . . is not hydrofluoric acid . . . It is the solid salt of sodium fluoride or sodium silico-fluoride which produces this effect. And it is not the same as that in the smog at all.

And then we have the physicians and dentists of Palo Alto, headed by Russell V. Lee, M.D., who lent their names to the statement that "The average five-year-old [in Palo Alto] has over three decayed *permanent* teeth." (Italics mine.)[69]

Outstanding even in such company, is A. P. Black, Ph.D., a chemist from the University of Florida. He calls himself the "father of fluoridation," and, together with Dean, engineered the endorsement by the American Water Works Association.

He told the American Dental Association that to give everyone in a community a lethal dose of fluoride, it would be necessary to add 40 tons of sodium fluoride to each million gallons of water. Such water would actually contain more than a lethal dose in each pint (4.54 grams), which seems like more than might be required. And besides, no one except Black was talking about doses which would kill you dead in your tracks. The point at issue is the cumulative effect of small daily doses over a long period of years, or a shorter period in sensitive persons. And if such use shortens your life by months or years, as it well may, who is to say that the dose is any less lethal because it took years instead of hours to kill?

It was also Black who told the Florida State Board of Health[70] that many chemicals are used in the treatment of water, and that most of these, if taken in the same (massive) doses that you would have to take of fluorides to produce death, would likewise produce death.* [71]

He admitted that he had no expert knowledge of medicine, dentistry, or the biological effects of fluoride, but this has never interfered with his making statements such as these. But, in his own field, he was no better.

He said that because all fluoride ions are alike, their actions will be the same, regardless of what else may be present, and that the Law of Mass Action does not apply at the concentrations found in potable waters. (This, in case you have forgotten your physical chemistry, is like saying that the laws of gravity do not apply to feathers.)

No chemistry professor should be making statements such as these, and when they do you should wonder why.

You may wonder less when you know that he serves frequently as a "water-works consultant," and is handsomely paid for reports in which his policy is to recommend fluoridation. Also, that members of his immediate family sell the chemicals and equipment he recommends.[72]

* In case the falsity of this is not obvious, I might mention that Benjamin Nesin, M.C.E., Director of Laboratories of the Department of Water Supply, Gas and Electricity of the City of New York, who probably knows as much about water supply toxicology as any man alive, has said: ". . . never in the history of water supply has a substance so toxic in nature, . . . and associated with so much adverse evidence affecting the public health, been considered seriously for introduction into the public water supply. . . . The proposal strikes at the very foundations of safe water supply practice and well-established concepts of factor of safety."

Conclusions

From all this, we can safely conclude:

(a) That fluoridation is not to be recommended.

(b) That science should be left to scientists.

(c) That those who call themselves scientists should refrain from endorsing quackery.

(d) That subsidies are not conducive to sound scientific conclusions.

(e) That the safeguards of traditional procedure are not lightly to be discarded.

(f) That we need to look more closely to our Constitutional rights and those of our fellows.

PART $\boxed{2}$

FLUORIDE POISONING IN THE FLUORIDATED CITIES

BY G. L. WALDBOTT, M.D.

GEORGE L. WALDBOTT, M.D.

Dr. Waldbott was born Jan. 14, 1898, in Speyer, Germany. He was graduated in 1921 from the University of Heidelberg, Germany, with the degree of M.D., and came to this country in 1924. He is a Fellow of the American College of Physicians, the American Academy of Allergy, the American College of Chest Physicians and the American College of Allergists. He is a former President of the Michigan Allergy Society, a former Vice-President of the American College of Allergists and an honorary member of several European allergy societies. He has published more than 125 medical papers, most of them original research. He founded and, at one time, directed allergy clinics at the Children's Hospital, Harper Hospital, Grace Hospital and St. Mary's Hospital in Detroit, Michigan. Among his notable contributions to medical literature is the first complete fungus survey to be made in the United States, the first report of a death from penicillin, the first article on Smokers' Respiratory Syndrome, now recognized as a common disease due to smoking. He is credited with the first pollen count and pollen survey made in Michigan, and is the author of a series of publications on allergic shock. Dr. Waldbott made some important contributions to the development of the technique of pollen treatment in hay fever. He also introduced bronchoscopic lavage as a life-saving measure in asthma. In his book on Contact Dermatitis he devised a new approach in determining the causative agents of this disease. He has published and has now in press, in medical journals, articles[1] about his original research on fluoride poisoning from drinking water.

Incipient Fluorine Intoxication

from Drinking Water

ANIMALS that have been inhaling fumes and grazing near aluminum, steel and fertilizer plants from which fluorine emanates, exhibit the following manifestations of chronic fluoride intoxication: They become lifeless and thin, their coats become coarse; they lie down and get up with difficulty; they limp and stand with curved, stiff backs and stiff hindquarters; swellings appear at the joints, exostoses on ribs and bones of head and shoulders.[1,2,3] In the young, the teeth become mottled; later they develop brown and black stains.

This disease has been adequately described by Roholm[4] in his classical monograph on fluorine intoxication of humans from industrial sources. Most striking is the vague character and great variety of symptoms (Table 4); like chronic intoxication from other toxic chemicals, not a single organ appears to be exempt.

from damage. Humans and animals die of general cachexia ("wasting away") or of intercurrent disease rather than from damage to a specific organ.

TABLE 4

SYMPTOMS IN 68 CASES OF CHRONIC CRYOLITE POISONING

Reproduction of chart in K. Roholm's classical monograph on fluorosis, illustrating the wide variety of vague symptoms, which is not unlike other types of chronic intoxication.

GASTRIC SYMPTOMS, mainly acute (lack of appetite, cardialgia, nausea, vomiting) 80.9%

INTESTINAL SYMPTOMS, mainly chronic (disposition to diarrhea, constipation) 33.8%

SYMPTOMS FROM CIRCULATION OR RESPIRATION* (shortness of breath, palpitation, cough expectoration) . 51.5%

SYMPTOMS FROM BONES, JOINTS AND MUSCLES (feeling of stiffness, indefinite or localized rheumatic pains) . 35.3%

SYMPTOMS OF NERVOUS CHARACTER (tiredness, sleepiness, indisposition, headache, giddiness) 22.1%

SKIN SYMPTOMS (rash) 11.8%

The literature on intoxication from drinking natural fluoride water, ranging in concentrations from two to sixteen parts per million, concerns itself mostly with bones and teeth.[5] In some areas, universal mottling or dental fluorosis with bone and joint involvement is encountered in the population. The major changes are hardening of bones, lime deposits in ligaments and tendons and exostosis of bones. In most of these studies, relatively little

---

* These patients were exposed to inhalation as well as ingestion.

attention has been given to symptoms attributable to damage in other organs.

In a more recent paper, Rao described what appears to be one of the major features of this disease, namely, partial palsy in arms and legs from drinking fluoride water at 7.2 parts per million.[6] In acute fluorine poisoning, this is recognized as a major clinical feature. Instability of gait, first reported by Lyth,[7] has been attributed to nerve damage of central origin or to the impingement of new bone substance upon the nerve at the exit from the spinal column. Rao also mentions disturbances of the lower urinary tract in his case. This observation has recently gained added significance by the observations of Herman[8] and Spira[9] that eight out of ten kidney stones from individuals living in nonfluoride areas contain relatively large amounts of fluorine (as much as 1500-1700 parts per million).

In another recent article, Frada and Mentesana[10] point to the high incidence of gastro-intestinal symptoms which were first described in animals by Leake and Ritchie.[11] Gastric pain, bloating in the abdomen and diarrhea alternating with constipation were noted. Skeletal changes demonstrable by X-ray were noted in only 45 percent of their cases with advanced fluorosis. Even in advanced experimental fluorosis in animals, such changes are detectable by X-ray in only a limited number of instances.[12]

Hearing disturbances were recently reported by Siddiqui[13] in seven out of thirty-two cases with crippling fluorosis from fluoride-water at concentrations ranging from 2.5 to 11.8 parts per million. Spira[14] was first to describe hearing defects in addition to brittle and spotted nails.

All authors agree that the clinical picture of chronic fluorosis in endemic areas is extremely complex.

Two fatalities from drinking natural-fluoride water are reported: one by Linsman and McMurray[15] of a twenty-two-year-old soldier with a cystic kidney who had lived for seventeen years in areas where the water contained fluorides varying in concentration from 1.2 to 5.7 parts per million. The description of this fatality strongly indicates that its cause was not the kidney disease, but general cachexia as described by Roholm in chronic industrial fluorosis.

The other case, a twenty-three-year-old individual in Argentina, died from drinking water containing fluoride at about two parts per million "and above." [16]

In all these reports, the diagnosis was based mainly on the changes in the bones and joints which occur only in the advanced stage of this disease, after prolonged consumption of fluoride water. No information on the incipient stage of this disease, which would make it possible to establish an early diagnosis, can be found in the literature.

A case presenting presumptive evidence of incipient chronic fluorine poisoning from drinking water at one part per million was described by me in 1955.[17]

After three years of drinking artificially fluoridated water at one part per million, this patient developed the following manifestations: severe backache in the lower spine, severe abdominal pain, nausea and marked flatulence after drinking water, mouth ulcers, pain and numbness in arms and legs and partial palsy in arms, extreme exhaustion and mental deterioration, beginning changes in the retina and hemorrhage from the bladder. Thorough laboratory and X-ray studies were entirely negative except that the blood-calcium level was slightly increased (11.6).

Nine competent consultants agreed that the patient was seriously ill, ruled out other diseases, but could not diagnose her case. The diagnosis was suggested by the complete subsidence of symptoms following elimination of fluoridated water and its recurrence upon its resumption; furthermore, by the close resemblance to the clinical picture of chronic fluorosis as described by Roholm and others and to what has been observed in animals.

A familial tendency to dental fluorosis was noted which might have predisposed the patient to the present illness. The patient's two children have a mild degree of mottling; she, herself, having resided in a fluoride area during childhood, has mottled teeth.

During two years of additional observation the patient has

been in perfect health, except for slight asthma at the height of the ragweed season in 1955.

On June 11, 1956, the 24-hour urinary output of fluoride, which had been 1.38, was .1 mg. (Normal in nonfluoride areas is .1 to .5 mg.)

On October 11, 1955, she was given an injection into the skin of 1/10 cc. of a 1:100 solution of sodium fluoride (1 milligram) of the same concentration. The fluoride tests reacted two plus. Within a half hour of the injection, a red streak developed along the arm from the site of the injection leading toward the lymph glands in the armpit. The patient complained of numbness in her fingers, legs, and hands, especially the little-finger area (ulnar nerve), and of a frontal headache which reached its climax after about four hours; it lasted 48 hours. This was accompanied by general malaise; there were no other symptoms. A few days later she was given a similar test with saline (salt) solution, with no effect whatsoever.

On August 15, 1956, she was given 15 mg. of sodium fluoride in 300 cc. of water on an empty stomach, in order to determine the urinary fluoride excretion. She was not aware that the water contained fluoride. Within ten minutes her face became flushed and she developed a severe attack of typical migraine headache associated with marked nausea, a sensation of flashing lights in both eyes, and pain in her arms and legs. This was followed shortly by diarrhea and cramplike pains in the lower abdomen. Throughout the day the patient was in a semicomatose state, and for three more days felt "dazed." She noted multiple bruises (suffusions) on her body and a swelling of salivary and parotid glands,* features which had been present during her illness two years previously.

In this reproduction of the symptoms of this disease without the patient's knowledge, one of the main requirements of scientific proof that her illness was a case of fluoride poisoning was fulfilled.

An apparently identical clinical picture was observed in a second hospitalized case, a 30-year-old woman. One of the con-

---

* These glands are known to eliminate fluorides from the body.

sultants at first suspected, but later ruled out, hyperparathyroidism and hyperventilation tetany, conditions which closely resemble those of fluoride poisoning.

The blood calcium was at the upper limit of normal 11.2; the urine calcium increased (393 milligrams).

This patient remained completely well upon drinking and cooking with distilled water. In August 1955 she was obliged to use city water again. Within one day, her muscle pains and intestinal symptoms returned. Further follow-up of this case is under way at this writing.

On November 21, 1954, eleven persons in Saginaw, Michigan, whom I interviewed, described the same syndrome.[18] They had improved considerably or were completely cured after the three-week interval since fluoridation had been discontinued in Saginaw. Restriction of motion in the lower spine and brittle nails were objective findings still evident at this time. Several patients had not been aware that fluoridation was in any way connected with their disease until after they had become well. There were more than twenty-five cases with bladder, joint and stomach symptoms which I disregarded because at that time I did not associate this condition with the disease; judging from recent observations, this might conceivably have been due to the fluoridated water.

The following is the history obtained in a typical case:

Case #19. Mrs. H.M., age 49, of Saginaw, Michigan, had lived as a child near Toronto, where the well water was said to contain fluorine. Her brother, sister and mother had "gray teeth" and "back trouble." She, herself, had suffered from "rheumatism" until she moved away at the age of nineteen. Subsequently, she had been in perfect health until 1947 when a uterine malignancy was removed.

During July, 1953, two years and three months after Saginaw had fluoridated its water supply, she noted a peculiar gnawing sensation in her stomach after eating, "as though there was something burning inside." Simultaneously, there was increasing stiffness and pain in the spine, relieved somewhat by using a board in her bed. The hands began to tingle in the areas about the fourth and fifth fingers; when peeling potatoes she was unable to finish. She lost control of her legs, which "seemed to collapse" under her. Gradually, she developed severe muscular pains in arms and legs. Throat, eyes and nose became extremely dry; the more she drank, the thirstier she became. Her head became "foggy," her thinking, "not clear"; the fingernails brittle and ridged; the hair began to fall out.

On hot days, the general weakness, mental sluggishness and dryness of the throat was especially enhanced. Because of greater consumption of water at this time, she began to suspect that drinking water aggravated her condition. On October 19, 1953, she started to use bottled water for drinking and distilled water for cooking. Within a few days her illness began to clear up; the pain in the stomach and dryness in the mouth improved first; the backache and muscular pains lasted for about three more weeks; the nails became normal after several months. She has been in perfect health since.

For further orientation about this disease, data were gathered by means of questionnaires from patients in various parts of the country who appeared to be affected by the same disease. The history thus obtained was considered especially significant because objective findings at this stage of the disease are very sparse. Replies to the questionnaires were carefully screened, supplemented by follow-up information from the patients, from hospitals and attending physicians. Whenever emotional factors appeared to be dominant, reports were scrupulously eliminated.

The following is a typical case:

Case #35. Mrs. T., age 53, of a West Virginia town, partook of fluoridated water from spring, 1954 until May 7, 1955.

According to one hospital report, Feb. 22, 1955, her main complaint was backache. On previous admissions, X-rays had shown a poorly functioning gall bladder and an ulcerated cervix which proved to be benign.

After November, 1954, there was gradually increasing soreness—no sharp pain, but more or less continuous ache in the lumbosacral region and between the shoulder blades. Stiffness in back and other joints, most marked on awakening in the morning, improved somewhat with activity.

Objective findings were: limitation in motion and some tenderness of the mid-dorsal and lumbosacral spine. The gall bladder was not visualized on cholecystography. Chest and spinal X-rays were normal. The dorsal and lumbosacral spine revealed minimal degenerative changes. The sedimentation rate was "elevated," blood sugar 60.

On April 21, 1955, physical examination at another hospital showed "tenderness practically everywhere," a questionable left sciatic tenderness, blood pressure 170/90, sedimentation rate 38.

With no definite cause for the muscular pains, she was treated for gout without success. A psychiatrist ruled out a psychosomatic origin of her condition.

Three weeks after fluoridation had been discontinued in mid-May, 1955, the symptoms showed marked improvement. They subsequently subsided completely. The patient first became aware that her case fitted the description of incipient fluorine poisoning several weeks after her recovery. She furnished the following supplemental information:

She had been allergic to certain drugs, including sulfa. When the backache started, she simultaneously developed a dull frontal headache. She was especially aware of weakness in her arms when lifting things. The muscular pains, limited at first to the lower spine and shoulder blades, had gradually affected her whole body down to her knees. Since about November 1, 1954, the pains had become so severe that she could no longer bend over, stoop or do housework. Her nails became brittle and tended to break. She developed visual disturbances; was surprised that she could see neither with nor without glasses. She had become forgetful, unable to concentrate and mentally sluggish.

Fluoridation was discontinued in her community on May 7, 1955. On the following October 17, the patient reported "perfect health."

In contrast to the previous cases, who showed symptoms of fluoride poisoning, the following one showed evidence of allergy to fluorides.

Case #25. Mrs. W.E.A., age 61, of Memphis, Tenn., with a personal and family background of allergy, had always been in good health except for occasional episodes of cystitis and a tendency to allergic nasal disease.

In April 1953, during a visit to Richmond, Va., she developed, within a few hours after arrival, nasal congestion, nasal discharge, swelling of the eyes associated with hives, and spastic pain in the upper abdomen. This was followed by severe diarrhea and flatulence. There was an intense feeling of general debility. Within two days after her return to Memphis, these symptoms cleared completely.

During a second visit to Richmond extending over a week (Oct. 1953) this condition recurred, again dominated by extreme general malaise and, in addition, by intense perspiration.

Other episodes occurred: one in January 1954, while on a four-to-five-day visit to Washington, D. C., and on two subsequent visits; one to Washington, D. C., in April 1954, the other to Richmond in August 1954. The last time the patient suffered excruciating pain in the stomach area and in the lower bowels which obliged her to be bedridden throughout the seven-day visit. Marked nasal congestion and discharge, burning pain on urination and frequency accompanied the condition.

At this time, it was first brought to her attention that both Richmond, Va., and Washington, D. C., were using fluoridated water. Upon the advice of a physician, she therefore restricted her fluid intake to bottled water and milk, strictly avoiding foods cooked with water. By taking charcoal tablets, antihistaminics and much milk, she was able to extend her trip to a period of ten days during which most of her symptoms subsided. After her return to Memphis the diarrhea and exhaustion persisted for another three days.

During another visit to Washington, D. C., in April 1956, she strictly avoided all food cooked with water, drank orange juice, milk and coffee made with bottled water exclusively. Upon brushing her teeth with a tooth paste she had been using for many years, she inadvertently rinsed her mouth with city water. Shortly thereafter a general soreness and itching in the mouth developed, followed within three days by ulceration of the oral lining. Upon again using bottled water for a mouth rinse, the condition cleared within four to five days. Ten days later it recurred when she intentionally rinsed her mouth with city water in Richmond, Va., in order to determine to her own satisfaction whether or not fluoride water was the cause of this latest episode of stomatitis.

At my suggestion an allergist in Memphis made the following studies on this patient:

On Feb. 21, an intradermal test with a 1:1000 dilution of 1 percent sodium fluoride sterilized by filtration, another with a 1:100 dilution were negative; control tests with 1:100 and 1:10 horse serum reacted negatively. No difficulties resulted from any of these injections. A patch test with 1 percent sodium fluoride was negative after forty-eight hours.

On Feb. 23 she was given an intradermal injection of 1/20 cc. of a dilution of 1:100 1 percent sodium fluoride in horse serum. This produced no reaction. The 1:10 dilution, however, induced some local itching within a few minutes and a generalized itching within twenty-four hours. This patient experienced diarrhea, swelling of both eyes, considerable nasal obstruction.

Several days later she was again tested with 1:10 horse serum intradermally with no local reaction and no generalized effect.

Since the patient felt that sources other than fluoride may have entered into the reaction of Feb. 23, the test with 1:10 sodium fluoride in horse serum was repeated on March 5 and again on March 23 with the same dosage; both times her nose became congested for three days, irritation of the bladder, gastric distress (pain, nausea, flatulence) and diarrhea occurred.

On July 14, 1956, the patient was examined in my office. This time a test with a 1:100 aqueous dilution of 1 percent sodium fluoride produced an itching flare reaction within ten minutes. Within two hours she developed gastro-intestinal symptoms, marked rhinorrhea, irritation in the throat which was followed by frequency of urination and pain in the bladder.

COMMENT: The presence of nasal symptoms concurrently with urticaria, gastro-intestinal and urinary manifestations strongly indicates that this reaction was allergic rather than evidence of intolerance to this drug. In other words, it was not true intoxication.

It is not unusual for an allergic reaction to be elicited by extremely small amounts of solution of a causative agent.

EVALUATION OF SYMPTOMS

So far, the evidence that this is fluorine poisoning is not final. It is based on the following facts:

1. The close resemblance to, if not full identity with, Roholm's description of industrial poisoning and with chronic fluorosis in animals. Changes in bones, joints and teeth cannot be expected in the incipient stage, as will be discussed later.

2. There is a parallelism of this disease with acute fluorine poisoning since mainly the same organs are involved, namely: muscles of arms, legs and back, the gastro-intestinal and the lower urinary tract.

3. The symptoms cleared upon eliminating fluoride water and recurred in those individuals who resumed it.

Further substantiating evidence is now being accumulated by reproduction of the disease with minute doses in patients who had completely recovered and by simultaneous fluoride excretion studies in these cases.

INCIPIENT VERSUS ADVANCED STAGE

In the incipient stage of this disease, two outstanding features of advanced chronic fluorine poisoning are absent, namely, demonstrable changes in bones such as increased bone density, coarsened trabeculation, increased thickening of the cortical bone, deposits of bone substance in ligaments and joints and mottled enamel. The latter occurs only in individuals who consume fluoride water while the teeth are developing, namely before the ages of ten or twelve.

The changes in bones, joints and ligaments, as a rule, do not develop within less than ten to thirty years of drinking fluoride water. Even in this advanced stage, roentgenological findings in bones and joints are not always present.

IS THERE A PSYCHOSOMATIC BASIS?

In order to rule out other diseases, adequate consultation by competent specialists was obtained in the hospitalized cases. They were unable to establish a diagnosis, but did not attribute the illness to psychosomatic causes.

This view is supported by the following facts: In two individuals subjected to exploratory surgery, the operation did not relieve the urinary symptoms or the abdominal pains.* An operation would certainly have produced a sufficient stimulus to reveal a psychosomatic basis. Months later these patients recovered completely without any treatment when fluoride water was eliminated without their knowledge. Other patients were aware neither that fluorides had been added to the drinking water nor that fluoridation had been discontinued. This, I believe is a more valid test than any carefully devised "blindfold" or placebo studies.

It is inconceivable that these patients could have been familiar with the description of this disease. Although residing in different parts of the country, they reported exactly the same symptoms in different words. For instance, the ulnar nerve damage is described in the following manner by a different person in each case: "cannot grip a golf club," "cannot peel potatoes," "cannot hold a hymn book in church," "cannot grip my steering wheel," "things are dropping from my grasp for no apparent reason."

The lack of control in their legs was described as follows: "my legs buckle under me," "I suddenly collapse," "my legs are not tracking," "my legs give way," "I suddenly lurch toward buildings."

---

* A third case in Lubbock, Texas, with natural fluorides at 4.2 ppm, with advanced skeletal fluorosis, the record of which I was able to study, had exploratory surgery which did not reveal the cause of an acute abdomen.

Examination Findings. Objective findings detectable on examination are: Limitation of motion in the spine; reduction of muscular power in arms and legs; ulceration of gums and stomatitis; brittle nails of fingers and toes; a restriction in the visual field (changes in the retina) and, according to Siddiqui,[19] hearing defects. Joint swelling and seborrheic dermatitis were present in some cases. Early X-ray changes are periosteal thickening and an increase in the markings of the trabecular bone structures.

Laboratory Data. Frada and Mentesana,[20] Siddiqui[21] and Murthi *et al.*[22] furnish information about laboratory data. There may or may not be a decrease in the red blood count and hemoglobin without abnormality of size or shape of the red cells; impairment of the kidney function (urea clearance test); a low acidity of the stomach (achlorhydria); a moderately high cholesterol; an increased sedimentation rate; a low basal metabolism; an increase in serum alkaline phosphatase.

In my own cases, increased urinary calcium output appeared to be a diagnostic feature. Disturbances in the electro-encephalogram of the type noted in calcium deficiency were observed. All other biochemical and hematological data in my cases as well as in those of the above-named authors were normal.

Symptoms of fluorine poisoning do not always parallel either fluorine levels in bones and blood, or its elimination in the urine. It is general knowledge that relatively large amounts may be stored and eliminated without ill effect.[23] Seven years, in one instance,[24] and even ten years after patients had stopped drinking fluoride water,[25] stored fluorine is still excreted in excessive amounts. On the other hand, there is evidence that relatively small doses can cause symptoms of poisoning in individuals or animals susceptible to the disease.[26, 27] The well-known authority on the subject, DeEds[28] observed that the "streaming through the system of fluorides, even in relatively small amounts, may cause considerable damage to the organs involved."

Urinary fluorine output depends mainly on the amount of stored fluoride mobilized from the bones under conditions not yet explained,[29] and on the amount of fluoride ingested in food, especially tea and fish. The absorption of ingested fluoride into the blood stream from the intestinal tract varies with the presence of other minerals in the water,[30] with the compound of the fluoride[31] and the acidity of the stomach.[32]

It is true such manifestations as the changes in bones, joints, ligaments, nails and hair are probably dependent on the amount of fluoride retained in these organs. However, symptoms originating in mucous membranes of the organs involved in ingestion and elimination of fluoride, such as the mucous membranes of the mouth (stomatitis), the stomach and bowels (gastritis and colitis), the lower urinary tract (cystitis, pyelitis) and skin, are not likely to be dependent on the amount of stored fluorine.

It is interesting to note that several patients started gastrointestinal symptoms within a few hours after ingestion of fluoridated water.

Clinical studies on fluorosis now in progress are designed to shed further light on this question. They also have already demonstrated the great impact which this whole subject may eventually have in the field of medicine.*

The following case of incipient arthritis is of interest since it suggests a close relationship of calcium excretion with fluorine output in urine in certain select cases of arthritis.

Mr. R.R., age 43, of Bloomfield Hills, Mich., developed signs of arthritis in finger joints and wrists without any other manifestations whatsoever. His well water contained 0.8 part per million of fluoride. On April 16, 1956, his 24-hour urine specimen contained 4.7 milligrams of fluorine (normal values in fluorine-free areas are .1 to .5 milligram); .705 gram of calcium (.050 to

---

* I have been assured by leading university professors in Switzerland, Germany, Spain, Italy, Poland, and Sweden that they will begin studies to corroborate my data.

.300 gram is considered normal; see Table 5). On April 23, during spontaneous improvement, the urine contained 1.82 milligrams of fluorine; .472 gram of calcium. On June 11, the patient was completely well. His urine specimen contained .69 milligram fluorine; .300 gram calcium for 24 hours.

TABLE 5

24 hr. Urinary Fluoride and Calcium Output of Mr. R. R., 43, with beginning arthritis in hands. (Well water contains .8 ppm fluoride)

DATE	FLUORINE	CALCIUM	SYMPTOMS
Apr. 16, 1956	4.7 mg.	.705 gm.	moderately severe
Apr. 23, 1956	1.82 mg.	.472 gm.	Spontaneous improvement
June 15, 1956	.69 mg.	.300 gm.	Changed to fluorine-free water Apr. 23
Aug. 10, 1956	1.26 mg.	.560 gm.	

Normal Fluorine content .1 to .5 mg. in fluorine-free areas; calcium .050 to .300 gm.

In this patient a generalized arthritis of moderate severity, lasting three weeks, was induced by a single dose of 15 milligrams of sodium fluoride in water.

In the following case, one symptom, namely ulcers in the mouth, dominated the clinical picture.

Mrs. A.P., age 49, was referred to me on January 21, 1956, for an allergic survey because of ulcers in the mouth (stomatitis). She had had frequent episodes of vague stomach disorders. Among the many unsuccessful therapeutic measures, she listed Vitamins C and B, extraction of all her teeth, radium treatment, mouth washes, disinfectants and Premarin therapy.

Tests for food sensitivity and a trial elimination of questionably reacting foods was unsuccessful.

On February 21, further history revealed that her condition started when she moved to her present home seventeen years ago. When away from home for two to three weeks, the lesions cleared completely. Since stomatitis constitutes a part of the syndrome described above, the water from the well which she had been using for the past seventeen years was analyzed: it contained 1.5 parts per million of fluoride.

A more detailed history with reference to incipient fluorine intoxication revealed a numbness in the ulnar nerve areas of both arms and fingers; considerable numbness in the legs, stiffness and pain in the lower spine; dull headaches involving the whole head, not related to eye strain or emotional upsets. The internist reported that gastro-intestinal X-rays did not explain the gastric pain and nausea after eating. A urologist had treated her for bladder disturbances to no avail. On March 19, 1956, a 24-hour fluorine determination of the urine showed 2.8 milligrams.

At a Detroit hospital the house officer recorded the following positive findings: several small coated ulcers on tongue, gums and cheek; submaxillary lymph nodes; a dry seborrheic skin lesion in the interscapular area; slight limitation of motion in the lower spine and tenderness in the lumbosacral joint; no abnormal reflexes. The X-ray showed destructive changes in the joint spaces between L5 and S1 and some evidence of spondylolisthesis.

Blood and urinary studies revealed nothing unusual except that the blood phosphorus was slightly increased (7.7 milligrams).

On March 19, 1956, the patient was told to discontinue using fluoride water for cooking and drinking. Two weeks later, the lesions in the mouth had disappeared completely for the first time in many years. The patient has been well since. Further studies are now in progress.

INDIVIDUAL SUSCEPTIBILITY

Tolerance to fluorides varies considerably among individuals. No estimate of the incidence of this disease can be made at this time. A highly individual susceptibility has been observed in chronic fluorosis in animals[33] and among different species of animals. Cattle, sheep and rats, for instance, are reported to be more susceptible than guinea pigs, chickens and dogs. Wilkie[34] and others observed a familial tendency to this disease.[35] Seven patients in my series have children whose teeth are mottled.

Factors linked with increased susceptibility to fluorosis are: malnutrition, old age, sex, dietary habits, additional exposure to fluorides through inhalation, absence of protective minerals (calcium and phosphorus) in food and water.

In chronic intoxication from trace quantities of other poisons such as lead, arsenic or beryllium, only highly susceptible individuals in a particular group of people may show symptoms. Statistical surveys are not likely to detect such cases.

Very little clinical information on chronic fluorosis is available in the medical literature in the United States. The observations above, like all new findings in medicine, require substantiation by others; yet they clearly point the way to a new avenue of clinical research which has heretofore been completely neglected and which conceivably can establish the source of a number of unexplained diseases. Results of further studies on the subject are now in press in several medical journals.

The Great Fluoridation

Promotion

THE U. S. Public Health Service is part of the Department of Health, Education and Welfare. Like the U. S. Army and Navy, its officers are under strict discipline and are obliged to obey orders from superior officers.

"Local Level Device." Mr. Oscar Ewing, Social Security Administrator, formerly in charge of the Public Health Service, in the foreword of the book, *America's Health* (Harper and Bros., publishers), known as America's ten-year health plan (1948-58), originated a carefully planned, highly effective device for introducing such measures as fluoridation: they should be decided on the local level. Indeed, one of the leading proponents of fluoridation present at the Hearings on H. R. 2341, in Washington, D. C., May 1954, was overheard to say, "That local level gimmick is the best thing we have."

State health officers and dentists have been instructed to emphasize this approach constantly. By urging city commissioners to make their own decision regarding fluoridation, the Public Health Service, as the central agency of the federal government, appears to have no part in it. Furthermore, lawmakers in Washington, D. C., stand aside because they are constantly being told fluoridation is not their affair; that it concerns local officials only.

Actually, a Public Health Service representative is usually "loaned" to the area from Washington for the purpose of stimulating the desire for fluoridation. Having accomplished his mission, he moves into other areas. Public Health Service federal tax money flows into these communities via the state health departments. Promotional material originates with public relations experts in Washington, D. C. Health officers work closely with officials of the American Dental Association.

"Scientific Propaganda." Fluoridation is a typical example of the way in which Public Health Service experts in public relations and in "social engineering" at the behest of top brass manage to convert highly controversial research findings into propaganda material for a "Public Health Measure." Every medical and dental society is guided on questions of public health by a Public Health Committee in which one or several health officials are accepted as the experts. These men, by virtue of the very nature of their jobs, are experts in the art of politics as well.

Public Health Service publications, for lay and scientifically-minded readers, have a wide circulation. Moreover, Public Health Service officials serve on editorial boards of most U. S. medical and dental journals in an advisory capacity. Practically all dental and medical schools depend upon Public Health Service grants-in-aid, from which salaries of deans and professors are paid. Dentistry became a part of the Public Health Service in 1948. As a result, Public Health Service officers are closely linked with the American Dental Association. Top health officers are salaried executives of the American Dental Association.*

* U. S. Public Health Service funds flow through state health departments to dental organizations. The dental organizations, in turn, use the

Indeed, such organizations as the American Public Health Association, the National Research Council, the American Association for the Advancement of Science are either largely composed of, or dominated by, Public Health Service officials. Health officials are represented on the Council of Pharmacy and Chemistry and the Council of Foods and Nutrition of the American Medical Association. Although they are composed mainly of eminent scientists, these councils rely entirely on evidence presented to them by health officials when they state they are not aware of harm from fluorides. Health officers are also active in the House of Delegates of the American Medical Association and the governing bodies of most state medical societies.

Officials of the American Medical Association have been automatically turning over all inquiries on the purely medical aspect of fluoridation to the Public Health Service or to the American Dental Association. As dentists, biochemists and statisticians, their experts have relatively little knowledge of the clinical aspect of fluoridation. However, these consultants bear impressive titles and through their interlocking memberships on boards and committees move in top scientific circles. Their influence on the distribution of government research money renders them highly desirable members in any scientific group, especially medical organizations. It is largely due to their personal influence rather than to their careful evaluation of scientific data that fluoridation has been endorsed by scientific societies.

THE OVER-ALL STRATEGY

Needless to say, the Public Health Service, the National Institutes of Health, as well as local and state health officials, are

---

funds to pay for promotional speeches by officials of the U. S. Public Health Service.

As an example of this, the financial report of the Maine State Dental Society of March 31, 1956, shows that the money which Dr. F. A. Arnold, Jr., Director of the Dental Institute of Health in Washington, D. C., received in payment for a lecture on February 24, 1955, came from the Public Health Service through the state health department. That is, the money was allotted by his close associates. According to Dr. Arnold's own statement in a letter to Mr. C. A. Barden of Oberlin, Ohio, dated August 16, 1956, as a government official he is not entitled to accept such fees.

held in highest esteem by citizens, officials and newspaper editors. Their publications and research data have always been considered a thoroughly reliable source of medical information. Personal opinions of health officials are, therefore, frequently accepted without question as though they were proven facts, even by physicians and scientists; few have felt obligated to examine critically the extensive and highly complex fluoridation literature.

In planning the over-all strategy for the promotion of fluoridation, the Public Health Service has relied heavily on this fact. Having first won the medical and dental professions for its cause, it could be expected that lay groups, especially the Parent-Teachers Association and the Junior Chamber of Commerce, would unhesitatingly fall in line.

The Document. This plan was clearly revealed in that amazing document, referred to by Dr. Exner on page 149: Proceedings of the secret meeting of dental state and territorial health officers in Washington, D. C., June 6-9, 1951.*

Incredible as it may sound, these men freely admitted that they knew nothing about the toxicity of fluorides at the so-called "safe" concentration, and relatively little or nothing about the effect of artificial fluoridation on teeth, since the two experimental studies, at Grand Rapids and Newburgh, were then far from completed. Yet with no evidence that fluoridation was safe and much to suggest that it wasn't, they laid plans for a promotional campaign of unprecedented scope, supported by tax money and Public Health Service prestige.

Characteristic of the casual manner in which problems of vital importance were handled is the following statement by Dr. Frank Bull of Madison, Wisconsin:

"This toxicity question is a difficult one. I can't give you the answer to it." Dr. Bull confessed himself equally baffled by the claim of critics that fluoridation is not needed: "They talk of other methods and when they get through adding up all the

---

* A copy of these minutes is in the possession of Mrs. A. R. Robinson, Seattle, Wash., and Mr. Rollin Severance, Saginaw, Mich. The correspondence and documentation as to how it was received are in the possession of Mr. Severance.

percentages of decay that we can reduce by such methods, we end up in a minus . . . when they take us at our own word, they make awful liars out of us."

Sentence First! Trial Afterward! Outside of Lewis Carroll's Wonderland, there is no precedent for the procedure followed by the Public Health Service in initiating and promoting the fluoridation program. The favorable results of the ten-year pilot-plant studies in Grand Rapids and Newburgh were apparently assumed in advance. By 1950 seventy-eight communities[1] had been encouraged to fluoridate their water systems, five of them as early as 1946; this, although in February of 1950 two of the chief promoters of the program, Dr. P. Jay of Ann Arbor, Michigan, and Dr. J. R. Blayney of Evanston, Illinois, declared publicly that no conclusive evidence of the effectiveness of fluoridation would be available until 1952.[2]

Between 1950 and 1952, no new, valid evidence arose to establish the safety of fluoridation. During those years public-health officials were still speaking of the "calculated risks" of the program. The few studies purporting to prove its safety all appeared later. Yet, in December of 1951, the American Medical Association announced its approval of the "principle" of fluoridation. Obviously this endorsement—not the findings of the pilot-plant studies, which still had four years to run—was all that was needed to trigger the all-out promotion of the program that immediately followed. Public-health officialdom felt confident now that lay and professional opposition must collapse in the face of such endorsement from on high.

How Scientists Are Won. Several methods have been employed by proponents to influence scientific groups and obtain the support of individual scientists:

1. The customary political buttonholing in a hotel or in club rooms prior to meetings in which important decisions are made.

2. Representing highly controversial data as scientific "facts."

3. Suppressing valid scientific research, both old and new, which tends to invalidate the proponent's case.

4. Making it extremely difficult for reputable scientists to present evidence against fluoridation.

Medical Societies. The American Medical Association endorsement was sponsored by two health officers, one from Connecticut, the other from Wisconsin, at the meeting of the House of Delegates in 1951. One of the Michigan delegates present at the initial meeting declared that he would have liked to oppose this measure. However, the vote was taken so precipitately that there was not even sufficient time for him to collect his thoughts, much less to inform himself adequately on the scientific aspects of the controversy. Another delegate didn't even know that the House had endorsed fluoridation.

Dr. Charles Farrell, Chairman of the Public Health Committee of the House of Delegates at the time, has described in detail the determinaton of the two health officials to force the issue through the House at a time when the delegates were not interested enough to study the project even if any reliable scientific data against fluoridation had been available.[3] In order to weaken the endorsement as much as possible, Dr. Farrell introduced the phrase "the principle of" and his substitute resolution passed the House.

A few key proponents hold high offices or are interlocking committee members in the professional organizations that have endorsed fluoridation.

In 1949, the American Water Works Association adopted its "permissive" endorsement of fluoridation. Its president at that time was A. P. Black, Professor of Chemistry at the University of Florida. Dr. Black has acknowledged that members of his family are president and vice-president of a company selling fluoridation equipment.[4] He has been active in the World Health Organization and was formerly a member of the National Dental Research Advisory Council which advises the Surgeon General concerning how to spend research money. He has been actively promoting fluoridation all over Florida and, among other things, was instrumental in getting Gainesville, his home town, to fluoridate as early as 1949 before any data respecting the pilot studies were available.

Dr. H. Trendley Dean, a high-ranking dental public health officer, is and has been a member of many committees of important research organizations. As former president of the Association for the Advancement of Science, he was chiefly instrumental in obtaining its endorsement. This organization wields a tremendous influence in scientific circles. Largely through his influence, St. Louis, the seat of his Alma Mater, Washington University, was persuaded to adopt fluoridation.

Manipulation of the local medical societies is much the same everywhere. The Public Health Committee of the society meets at the behest of the Health Commissioner. Its members are given one-sided literature exclusively extolling the great benefits and absolute safety of fluoridation. Some of the officers of the medical society receive detailed instructions on how to initiate promotion and how to discredit the opposition, which, they are told, is of no consequence.

When members of the public-health committee of a medical society in a Michigan town asked for more time to study the matter, the Health Commissioner stressed the urgent need for fluoridation and pressed for immediate action. This tactic prevents anybody from making the critical study of the evidence which might result in the rejection of the program.

Once an endorsement has been given, the governing members of the society feel obliged to maintain and actively defend their stand and the general membership assumes that their position is based on thorough study.

The experience of the Essex County Medical Society of Windsor, Ontario, is typical. A physician interested in presenting evidence against fluoridation was assured that he would be duly informed should the matter come up. That same week at the regular meeting of the society the Medical Officer of Health urged immediate endorsement. It was quickly passed before any evidence on the other side could be heard. A request for presentation to the society of cases of fluoride intoxication from drinking water was denied. Similar accounts from many cities have come to my knowledge.

Armed Services. Children under ten do not serve in the armed forces and only a comparative few of the servicemen stationed at our military bases are married men with families. Nevertheless, service men have no choice but to drink fluoridated water.

When asked why the Lakehurst Naval Station is fluoridated, in view of the meagre benefit that could accrue to servicemen, Dr. E. G. Ludlam, New Jersey State Dental Health Director wrote, in a letter to Mr. W. A. Hodges dated Feb. 10, 1956:

". . . Because it is well known that naval and military authorities are generally considered to be appropriately concerned about safeguarding the health of their personnel, the Department felt, upon being informed of the Lakehurst fluoridation, that this action might have a beneficial effect of furnishing another illustration of fluoridation to strengthen the efforts of those of us who would like to see controlled fluoridation more widely adopted in New Jersey." In short it seemed proper to waste military appropriations to promote adoption of a dubious civilian public health measure. The welfare of the service man and his children was clearly not the main consideration.

Health Departments. Mr. J. W. Shelmerdine, a member of the board of health of Hartford, Conn., stated in a letter to the *East Hartford Gazette* of August 9, 1956, that the Connecticut State Health Commission had received a grant of three million dollars from the U. S. Public Health Service for scientific research—on condition that the Commission would promote fluoridation in Connecticut.

MISREPRESENTATION OF SCIENTIFIC REPORTS

A scientist desiring to study fluoridation naturally turns for information to the Public Health Service or to the American Dental Association for literature. He receives a bundle of scientific and lay publications containing complicated graphs and charts as well as scientific reprints. A careful analysis of this material requires much time and great persistence since literally thousands of articles on the subject must be consulted.

Eventually the scientist discovers that summaries and conclusions of the many scientific publications which purport to show the safety of fluoridation do not correspond with what is indicated in the text, that much of the literature is based upon the wholly unproven hypothesis that fluorine is essential for healthy teeth.

One of the investigations most frequently cited to prove the safety of fluoridation is the Bartlett-Cameron study. This study shows severe damage to health in both cities. Yet the Public Health officers who made this study, as well as supporting members of the National Research Council, categorically assert that the damage noted in the population is of no significance.[5] One of the chief fallacies in this study is the fact that the drinking water of both cities contains fluorides and that no comparison was made with the over-all disease incidence in the United States.

In a subsequent article (part of the Bartlett-Cameron study) published in the *Journal of Roentgenology* (74:844-855, Nov. 1955) a series of twenty-one cases exhibiting bone changes is presented. In the conclusion it is implied that no other damage indicative of fluoride poisoning was found although the text itself presents only fragmentary data on three of the twenty-one cases. Even in these three cases, there is clear evidence that at least two individuals manifested additional symptoms of fluorine poisoning. Detailed information on the twenty-one cases was refused by Dr. N. C. Leone with the explanation that the X-rays were read by experienced roentgenologists (no one questioned this!) and that all the material was carefully reviewed by competent scientists.

Research Without Well-Established Premises. Elaborate and carefully executed studies are reported, the thoroughness of which is bound to impress scientists who accept in good faith the premises of these studies. Actually they are based on unproven assumptions. For example, urine studies were made of 900 children in Newburgh, New York.[6] After ten years of fluoridation, no albumin, casts or red blood cells, which are signs of kidney disease, were found. This, the authors assert, adds to the "mass of evidence" proving that fluoridation is safe. Actually these studies prove nothing. The experimental work on animals upon which this survey of children is based, clearly revealed that even in far advanced experimental poisoning, no casts, albumin, or red blood cells were found in the urine.[7] This is confirmed by several other reports and from personal correspondence with clinicians who have had actual experiences with fluoride poisoning in men.

Omission of Important References. Very rarely does one find reference in the proponent literature to the many publications reporting damage to animals and humans from fluoridated drinking water at or near the so-called safe concentration.[8] Such omissions are especially noticeable in the report by a committee of the St. Louis Medical Society which states that, "There is no published record of any injury to health of any person drinking naturally fluoridated water with a concentration as high as eight parts per million." Yet proponent scientists are now acknowledging that "crippling fluorosis" occurs from concentrations as low as two parts per million.[9] Because several scientists of high authority in other fields contributed to the St. Louis report, it has misled more physicians than any other proponent article concerned with the safety of fluoridation.

Several thorough studies on chronic fluorine poisoning by such noted authors as DeEds, Hart and Phillips, discussions on the subject by Hanzlik, Leake and Geiger[10] are completely ignored. The monumental research by Hans Borei[11] which included a review of existing literature on the effect of fluorides on enzymes is scarcely ever mentioned in this country. Anyone who reads it will unquestionably become greatly concerned about placing such a poisonous substance in drinking water. And yet Dr. Leona Baumgartner, the N. Y. Health Commissioner, who should be familiar with this work, ridicules any mention of the deleterious effect of fluorides on enzymes.

Borei's book, written before the fluoridation era, is now out of print. Its publishers stated in a letter to me, two years ago, that this was the case. But they later said, in a letter dated August 3, 1956, to Mrs. W. M. Sykes, Huddersfield, England, that they have no record of having published such a book. A copy of this book is in my possession. Strangely, its author, one of the greatest investigators on the subject, is now a member of the faculty of a university in the United States and has abandoned his original research on fluorides. He[12] declines to comment—as does Dr. DeEds[13]—on anything pertaining to fluoride poisoning on the grounds that he has made no further studies. Both authors are either employed by the federal government or receive Public Health Service research grants.

In Public Health Service publications, McClure's studies are quoted exclusively, whereas those by Wallace-Durbin and Muhler, whose research shows that even in the most minute doses fluoride accumulates in the system, are omitted.

Dr. H. C. Hodge and associates stated in the *Journal of Rheumatic Diseases,* 14:378, December 1955, that crippling fluorosis (i.e., *advanced* fluoride poisoning) occurs from drinking natural-fluoride waters at 2 to 16 parts per million. A few months later (March 1956), in the *Journal of the American Dental Association,* the same Dr. Hodge made the following statement: "It is obvious that crippling fluorosis can never be produced by drinking fluoridated water."

Scientific publications showing that fluoride ions behave differently when in company of other ions, especially calcium and magnesium, are rarely reported; the official line is propagated that "an ion is an ion" and there is no difference between artificially and naturally fluoridated water.

SUPPRESSION OF RESEARCH

The experience of Dr. Alfred Taylor, University of Texas, constitutes one of the most striking examples of how scientific information unfavorable to fluoridation is being suppressed. The following is quoted from a letter by Dr. Taylor to the writer:

> In a routine check of compounds for possible anticancer qualities, sodium fluoridated drinking water was given to mice in order to test the effect on the tumor incidence of a tumor strain of mice. The initial results, based on two

experiments, indicated a shorter life span in the mice drinking the treated water. The results of these two experiments were questioned by several fluoridation proponents. A series of ten more experiments were completed in which mice of another strain and a fluorine-free diet were utilized. As the attached paper shows, there has been completed a total of twelve experiments involving 645 mice. The discrediting attacks made on my research, which have been given wide publicity by the ADA, are based on my two preliminary experiments; the final results are completely disregarded.

There are two papers which are cited as discrediting my work. First, an investigation by Dr. Fleming of Harvard, who found that twenty parts per million fluoride, as NaF, inhibit the growth, to some extent, of cancer implants. As a general rule, any compound at a dosage toxic to the animal will have this effect.

The other paper was by Bittner and Armstrong. In their experiment, 36 mice received five parts per million, 34 mice ten parts per million fluorine, in their drinking water, and 31 mice served as controls. The results showed no significant difference in the age at which cancer developed. Since my data indicates that fluoridated water does not affect every mouse in a group, but only certain susceptible individuals, it becomes necessary to have large numbers of animals in order to obtain results which are not due to chance segregation. A control group consisting of 31 animals would be insufficient to reveal differences on the order of those encountered in the work here.

Rarely is reference made to experiments by Harris and Nizel who showed that food grown in areas high in minerals prevents tooth decay regardless of whether or not it contains fluorine; to the article by Weddle and Muhler, who set out to determine whether or not fluorine is necessary for good teeth and found no such evidence. Dr. Paul H. Phillips, in the *Journal of the American Dietary Association*, 32:110-114, Feb. 1956, shows that fluorine is not essential for production of good teeth.

When Public Health Service officials found that the natives

of Samoa[14] had perfect teeth without fluorides in water, their survey was not published.

When the University of Oregon showed that fluorine in food pellets caused death to a chinchilla herd, the money for these studies was quickly withdrawn by the Public Health Service, which had financed the investigation.[15]

When in Ottawa, Kansas, after three years of fluoridation, tooth decay in five- to six-year-old children doubled, the studies were dropped.

When evidence on decay in fluoridated cities, namely, Sheboygan, Wis., and Lewiston, Idaho, was found to be unfavorable to fluoridation, it was not made available.

Five years after the Grand Rapids experiment started, both the city adding fluorides and its control, Muskegon (fluoride-free), showed a reduction in dental caries in one age group.[16] Thereupon the control was abandoned. It was stated that the people of Muskegon demanded fluoridation in order that they should no longer be deprived of the benefits of this great discovery.

Attempts to Deny Clinical Data. In Evanston, Ill., fluoridated since 1946, a resident believed that she was suffering from fluoride poisoning. Dr. W. H. Tucker, health officer, asked by Miss M. M. to investigate her case, replied as follows: "As I indicated to you in my letter under date of November 2, 1954, one part per million of fluorine in drinking water has no harmful effect whatever, on any human being. This has been proven repeatedly by extensive medical research. Apparently your difficulties are due to some factor other than fluorine in the drinking water provided by the City of Evanston."

When the health officer of Highland Park, Michigan, Dr. James Nunn (Hearing before the Highland Park City Council Nov. 28, 1955), was informed about two cases of poisoning, the only step he took was to inquire among friends of the patients as to whether or not they were neurotic. He has recently attempted to investigate. The city is being sued for damages by one of these patients.

Valid scientific material is countered in the following way:

It is flatly stated that no physician in a particular fluoridated town has seen such cases. In Highland Park, Michigan, for example, every physician was asked the question, "Have you seen any cases of poisoning from drinking water?" Not knowing anything about the disease, or how to diagnose it, the physician naturally answers that he hasn't.

When the Public Health Service no longer can deny that valid data have become available against fluoridation, despite their efforts to suppress them, they resort to such subterfuges as the following, which appeared in a letter written by Dr. D. E. Price, Acting Surgeon General, to Congressman G. Canfield of New Jersey, dated May 31, 1956: ". . . the cases mentioned by him [Dr. Waldbott] have not been found reported in any of the numerous scientific publications *which we receive regularly.*"

Shouldn't an agency which is responsible for protecting the health of the nation obtain and evaluate all available data?

Medical Journals. How health officials as members of editorial boards virtually establish a censorship of scientific articles against fluoridation is shown by the following example:

The editor of a state medical juornal intended to publish the first report I had made of fluorine poisoning from artificially fluoridated water. The paper was first submitted to consultants; these were Public Health Service officials and dentists, not one of whom had done research on fluorine poisoning. Having decided against publishing it, the editor was courteous enough, upon inquiry, to provide his reason for this decision: A photostat of the Linsman-McMurray fatality report in which, by a typographical error, the fluorine content of the water was stated as 12 parts per million instead of 1.2 parts per million. The correction appeared a few months later in the same journal. By ignoring this correction, the consultant had managed to place doubt in the editor's mind regarding my integrity.

When the editor of the journal of an important medical society was asked whether an article I had prepared, entitled "Medical Evidence Against Fluoridation," could be considered for publication, he stated *without seeing the article* that he would be obliged to "consult the policy-making members" of the medical society first. This article was of sufficient scientific value to be subsequently published by two leading foreign dental journals, at their request.

Evasion of Debate. On numerous occasions, critiques of the proponent scientific data have been presented to the Public Health Service for a rebuttal. The Public Health Service either refrains from answering, or curtly dismisses the issue by referring to the "great authorities" who endorse fluoridation. Instead of dealing with the subject matter itself, they attempt to show that the author is not qualified to discuss matters relative to fluoridation. They constantly reiterate that the "evidence is outdated," or "quoted out of context."

THE A.D.A.'S PROPAGANDA TACTICS

In 1954 the American Dental Association published a pamphlet entitled, "How to Obtain Fluoridation for your Community." This pamphlet suggests promotional methods unprecedented in scientific history, not even rivaled by the high-powered promotion of a commercial product. Officially the Public Health Service does not attempt to interfere with the formation of opinion at the local level. Officially the service has no responsibility for the swarms of well-heeled promoters that have descended upon numerous cities and towns since the start of the fluoridation program.

Out of the blue a chemist or dentist arrives in town and starts propagandizing the Parent-Teachers Association, the Junior Chamber of Commerce, service groups, the local dental society. His mission accomplished, he moves to another town.

A dentist who had been the key promoter in Greenwich, Conn., appeared several months later in a California town. A key promoter in Louisville, Kentucky, turned up in Hawaii, where he devoted his entire time to promoting fluoridation. Similarly, a health officer who organized the fluoridation campaign in South Carolina was reported several months later to be the driving power in a California town. Some of these promoters are assigned or "loaned" by the Public Health Service, others are paid public-relations experts of the American Dental Association. In Florida, the Association pays a public-relations man an annual salary of $6500 for his services.

Silencing Opponents. This is not the first time that the policies and projects of the Public Health Service have been opposed by professional and lay critics. Never before, however, has the Service gone so far as to defame and attempt to silence its opponents.

In effect, this tactic of slander and intimidation is recommended in the American Dental Association pamphlet already referred to in which it is stated that "a critical examination of the opponent literature usually discloses this evidence to be documented from out of date materials written by well-known persons; obtained from little-known lay magazines, newspaper articles, 'letters to the editor,' or health faddist periodicals; based on incorrect or ill-chosen terminology used by well-known persons; partial quotes from authoritative sources; misinterpretations based on an incomplete knowledge of the subject; unwarranted or hasty conclusions drawn from research work; completely unsubstantiated and undocumented statements by obscure 'scientists'; and little known, or out of date, unrecognized medical and dental periodicals, dictionaries and encyclopedias."

Dentists. The American Dental Association has systematically stifled expressions of views of dentists opposed to fluoridation.

Section 20 of the American Dental Association Code of Ethics was adopted in 1950 obviously in order to forestall opposition to fluoridation. It prohibits American Dental Association members from taking a position publicly in a matter of education of the public unless the program has the approval of the dentists of a community or state "acting through the appropriate agency of the dental society."

Aware that this section interfered with the constitutional right of freedom of speech, the American Dental Association in October, 1955, toned it down to read as follows: "that such programs are in keeping with the dignity of the profession and the custom of the dental profession in the community." However, unless a dentist is willing to endorse blindly any statement of the American Dental Association, the dissident dentist must still expose himself to disciplinary action. There are several instances of censorship by the American Dental Association:

Two dentists in North Carolina have been expelled from the society for one year because they campaigned against fluoridation.

Dr. A. C. Baumann, a dentist in Cleveland, Ohio, stated:

"All sorts of attempts were made to insult me personally and to question my motives; insinuations and veiled threats with regard to Section 20 of the Code of Ethics—which inhibits dentists from making public utterances not in accord with the American Dental Association official position—were employed."

Dr. Max Ginns, of Worcester, Mass., was summoned to appear before the Ethics Committee of his dental society because he publicly opposed fluoridation.

John E. Waters, D.D.S., Coronado, California, was threatened with disciplinary action if a series of articles against fluoridation appeared under his name.

Dr. A. B. MacWhinnie of Seattle was denied the right to speak against fluoridation at his own dental society. When he submitted his viewpoint to his state journal (he had previously written editorials as a member of the publications committee), his editorial was removed at press time. He states: "If the profession is not qualified to discuss this question, then who is? With rigid censorship of all society-controlled dental journals it leaves the professional man no choice but to go directly to the public."

Laymen. If the opponent is a lay person, no matter how solid a citizen he may be, he is identified with one of three groups: "crackpots," "religious fanatics," or "those who have something else to sell." His friends, employer, and trade organization descend on him to make sure that he is properly "instructed."

In a Michigan town, a businessman lost much of his clientele because he opposed fluoridation. His customers were made to believe that he did not have the public interest at heart. In another Michigan town, an undertaker was "instructed" by the president of the local medical society that were he to persist he might lose the good will of the local physicians, an unpleasant prospect for an undertaker.

A radio announcer in Cincinnati, Ohio, was informed of his dismissal less than an hour after he had called an article in the *Daily Worker* promoting fluoridation, "the kiss of death to the fluoridation project."

Rev. Father W. J. Enright of St. Patrick's Rectory, Toronto, received a personal letter from the Director of Dental Services, Prince Edward Island, telling him that "clergymen should not interfere with such matters."

At the hearings of the Florida State Board of Health, August 20, 1955, everyone who attended was requested to sign his name and address. Subsequently, some of those who had opposed were warned by their employers to refrain from further activities of that sort.

Scientists. If the opponent happens to be a physician, it is pointed out that his opposition to fluoridation is shared by crackpots, chiropractors, Christian Scientists, naturopaths, faddists of all sorts. Therefore, it is implied he belongs to the same group. If he is a journalist he is called "a crank" or "sensational."

Dr. H. E. Hilleboe, New York Commissioner of Health, has stated on several occasions that "those who oppose fluoridation are cultists or faddists, uninformed or misinformed."

Dr. George F. Lull, Secretary of the American Medical Association, refers to opponents as "unscrupulous."

Dr. Haven Emerson calls them "nitwits."

When a physician opposes fluoridation, the local dental society requests his medical society to censure him. Such a request was made to the Wayne County Medical Society in my own case. In Dayton, Ohio, seven physicians received summonses to appear before their society. It is to the credit of these medical societies that no action concerning censorship was taken.

In Detroit, several opposing physicans have had personal visits from a local dentist for the purpose of "instructing" them regarding the medical (!) aspect of fluoridation. His only equipment for this action was the American Dental Association's promotional material.

After the medical and dental societies are won by the State Health Department under guidance by the Public Health Service and with the help of federal tax money, the local citizenry is indoctrinated.

Emotions of citizens are aroused by means of photographs of babies appearing in the daily papers implying that without fluoridation they would be deprived of their just due. Some newspapers point to the injustice being perpetrated against youngsters who, because of being below voting age, cannot make their desires known. The Parent-Teachers Association and the Junior Chamber of Commerce take the lead in supporting the project. The former is highly responsive to emotional appeals for the good of the children. The latter organization by its very nature is interested in furthering any move that promotes business. The chemical and sugar industries have a strong influence on this group.

Most reprehensible of all is the use of the local welfare agency to sell this so-called panacea to the community as a project worthy of private donations. Thus welfare funds combine with tax supported grants-in-aid and corporation money to promote fluoridation.

Most of the time it is not necessary to organize such broadspread support. Fluoridation has been introduced quietly by a few dentists, a health official, plus a few Parent-Teachers Association women. They invite members of the city councils to dinner or cocktail parties. Before the dessert is served, the decision to fluoridate their town has been made.

Representative Delaney states that this is the customary procedure by which U. S. Congressmen are won for the cause. Even the mayor of a town may not know that his town is fluoridated (Tuckahoe, N. Y.). In many communities, the citizens were not told that fluoridation had been introduced until weeks or months after the deed was accomplished; then it appeared in their newspapers in fine print.

The Press. It has been alleged that some of the violent pro-fluoridation newspapers are influenced because of revenue from advertising by chemical corporations, sugar and soft drink industries. This is not likely, especially with respect to large metropolitan newspapers, several of which have opposed the program. Magazines are more vulnerable to the pressure of advertisers.

It is significant that except for *Harper's, The Freeman, The New Leader, The National Review, Mercury* and *Coronet* no magazine of large national circulation has been willing to publish an article critical of fluoridation. In the case of *Coronet*, its publication of James Rorty's pro-and-con article was followed by an inexplicable refusal to permit the use of reprints.

Interested Industries. How does one explain the haste, the suppression of evidence, the intimidation and slander of opponents, and the unscrupulous propaganda that have characterized the promotion of the fluoridation program?

Is professional zeal, added to the drive for expansion which the Public Health Service shares with other government agencies, enough to explain conduct which is equally unbecoming to scientists and to public servants and which is unprecedented in the history of public health administration in this or any other country?

Without attempting to answer these questions it may be noted that commercial interests outside the Public Health Service and the American Dental Association stand to benefit substantially from the fluoridation program, and that these interests have exerted themselves powerfully to bring about its adoption. Sodium fluoride and sodium silico-fluoride are made from waste products of the aluminum, fertilizer and steel industries. The price of sodium fluoride has increased greatly since 1945. New plants are being built throughout the country to satisfy the increased demand. Even before the public health service gave the green light, the fluoride manufacturers had begun advertising their products in the *Journal of the American Water Works Association* and in the trade press of the chemical industry. The same manufacturers have helped to finance the fluoridation research of foundations and university departments which have supported their program. Such grants were made by the TVA, a major government producer of fluorides, by the Aluminum Company of America, and by the Permanente Metal Corporation, to the Kettering Institute and the University of Cincinnati. These grants stipulate that all research reports be submitted to the industrial sponsor "for criticism and suggestion" prior to publication.[17]

Thus, Dr. F. F. Heyroth, Assistant Director of the Kettering Laboratory, was required to submit to Alcoa and other industrial sponsors his article entitled, "Toxicological Evidence of the Safety of Fluoridation of Public Water Supplies." The article turned out to be an incredibly biased and selective review of the literature, embodying flagrant misquotations as well as inexplicable omissions.

In the heat of the battle in Birmingham, Ala., Mr. H. A. Lilly wrote four letters to the papers—two to the *News* and two to the *Post-Herald*—strongly urging fluoridation. He gave his name and address, of course, but did not mention that he was manager of the Aluminum Company of America branch there, a company which sells sodium fluoride or its equivalent for city water supplies.

PART 3

THE FLUORIDATION-RESISTANCE

MOVEMENT

BY JAMES RORTY

The Water Engineers

Know Their Subject

AN essential stroke in the strategy of the proponents of fluoridation was the neutralization of the water engineers. This task was assigned to Dr. A. P. Black, a professor of chemistry at the University of Florida. Dr. Black's ardent promotion of fluoridation on the expense account, for travel at least, of the Public Health Service has greatly aided the commercial activities of his son, who sells fluoridating equipment.

At a convention of the American Water Works Association, Dr. Black, with the help of H. Trendley Dean, representing the Public Health Service, managed to obtain passage of the permissive resolution which the Public Health Service and the American Dental Association have falsely represented as an "endorsement" of fluoridation.

The fact is, the resolution declared merely that water

departments and companies might properly participate in a fluoridation program "in communities where a strong public demand had developed [we have seen how such "demands" are artificially created] and the procedure has the full approval of the local medical and dental societies, the local and state health authorities, and others responsible for communal health."

Among those clearly responsible for communal health are, of course, the water engineers themselves, including those engaged exclusively in water plant design, as well as those engaged in plant operation. Their responsibility is in fact far greater and more immediate than that of the dentists or the physicians. Moreover, the water engineers cannot afford to take this responsibility lightly, if only because their reputations and their jobs are at stake; if anything goes wrong they will be first to get the blame. Realizing this, the water engineers equip themselves with far more training, knowledge and experience in the field of water toxicology than the average physician or dentist; more, in fact, than is possessed by a good many health officers.

Fluoride pollution from industrial wastes is and has been for many years one of the recognized environmental hazards against which the water engineer must protect the public or private water system for which he is responsible. In areas where the natural fluorine content of the ground water is high it has frequently been his task to find fluorine-free water sources, or to devise economical methods of defluoridating the existing supply.

Hence the astonishment and alarm with which experienced water engineers regarded the launching, in 1950, of the Great Fluoridation Promotion. As water toxicologists they had read the literature of fluoride poisoning. They knew, despite the reassuring assertions of the Public Health Service's experts, that this literature was full of reports showing damage to human health from water containing fluorine at only a little more than the recommended one part per million level. As water engineers, they knew, with respect to all such highly toxic chemicals, a fiftyfold margin of safety is customary and necessary. They knew, further, that it would be utterly impossible for them to maintain even a tenfold safety factor if they were forced to introduce into the water mains the notorious "bad boy of the halogens": a corrosive chemical so destructive of transmission, distribution, and service equipment that maintenance would thenceforth become an expensive and nerve-wracking nightmare, with the possibility of an epidemic of fluoride poisoning always in the background.

They knew this because it was their business to know it, and many of them thought it was their business to explain it when the fluoridation program was first proposed to the city authorities who employed them. In some cases their influence was sufficient to prevent the adoption of the program. In others they were brushed aside by mayors and councilmen who were unable to believe that the Public Health Service would sanction the program without exhaustive evidence to prove fluoridation was safe, and who were themselves ill equipped to evaluate the massive evidence which proves it isn't.

In St. Louis, the opposition of the water departments was overcome with difficulty. In New York, Commissioner Arthur C. Ford and his aide, B. C. Nesin, director of the department's laboratory and one of America's leading water toxicologists, have successfully opposed repeated efforts by the New York Health Department to bring about adoption of the program. In April of 1956, Commissioner Ford issued the following statement setting forth his department's position with regard to fluoridation of the New York City water supply system:

> Under the City Charter, the Commissioner of the Department of Water Supply, Gas and Electricity is charged with the responsibility of maintaining the purity and wholesomeness of the city water supply. The matter of purity has a direct bearing on the people and involves the determination and evaluation of the tolerance of suspect, hazardous or toxic substances which may, in some manner, gain access to the water supply. Fluoride is a toxic substance.
>
> The department has extensive laboratories staffed by reputable scientists and competent sanitary engineers, with a massive library in which is contained over five thousand references on the subject of fluorine alone. We have con-

tinued to study and evaluate the effect of toxic substances as related to water supply. The matter of fluorides has been under our scrutiny for over twenty years.

The addition of fluorides to the water supplies is not coupled with the concern of maintaining or improving the quality of the water or making it safe. No one has suggested that dental caries is a water-borne disease nor that water is the cause of dental decay. No satisfactory reason has ever been advanced to show why everyone in a community must be compelled to risk life-long extraordinary exposure to the toxic action of fluorides, particularly when safer, more effective and more economical ways of administering fluorides for caries reduction in children's teeth have been pointed out and are available.

Whatever the merits of fluoridation, it would not concern us as a department if the question of water supply safety were not involved. But we are concerned and our concern is primarily with the safety of the water supply for each and every individual of our entire population of eight million people throughout the city.

We are aware that the fluorides are extremely toxic substances and evidence exists to show that even at the recommended level of one part per million of fluoride in drinking water, people in fluoridated communities have been harmed. A very small percentage among a population of eight million, sensitive to the chemical and adversely affected, would constitute a seriously significant number of persons harmed.

We know of reputable, independent medical authorities throughout the United States and in the local area who have found evidence of fluoride damage to persons living in fluoridated communities. These medical authorities disagree with the fluoride hypothesis, and they have raised grave questions with respect to the safety of the procedure for an entire population which includes the young, the old, the susceptible, and the infirm as well as the healthy.

No one has made a claim that the ingestion of fluoride can be of benefit to the teeth beyond the formative years of childhood. Because of this, and for reasons of safety and economy, this department has proposed that the City distribute fluoride tablets through health stations, free of charge, for parents to administer to children. The cost to the City, ascertained at less than 25 cents for a thousand days for each child, would be less than one fifth of the cost of a fluoridated water program. Tablets (a pharmaceutical grade in contrast with the commercial by-product used in water fluoridation) would provide an exact procedure, under control, to be taken only by those during the formative period of their teeth.

Fluoride, besides being a toxic substance, is not all excreted when taken into the system, a significant percentage remaining cumulatively. Fluoridation of the drinking water at any level of concentration is a very indiscriminate procedure since children drink widely varying amounts of water, each according to taste, physical activity, and seasonal variations of the year. The daily intake of one child often differs greatly from that of another who may drink milk, fruit juices and soft drinks in abundance.

How, then, will each child receive his appropriate share of fluoride when each drinks widely differing amounts from the same source of water having a given concentration in parts per million of fluoride?

The problem of managing the control of dosage of fluoride chemical to obtain uniformity throughout a grid-work of more than 5,000 miles of pipe and tunnels involving different sources and pressure gradients, as in the New York system, is formidable. None of those who have made statements to the contrary has ever had the experience nor do they possess knowledge of what the exact result would be. Our concern and responsibility in the department is to provide the people of our city with a dependable supply of the purest and safest water possible. No one can guarantee similar safety to all the people in the City of New York under a program using the water supply as a fluoride vehicle.

Unfortunately the forum on the subject of fluoridation is not as open as it should be, even among professions. There has been too much of emotion, blind following, and lack of objective thinking by too many people on both sides of the question.

The people of the City of New York are entitled to know the risks they are being asked to assume before endorsing a program involving so many questions yet unanswered.

Arthur C. Ford
Commissioner

Damage to Equipment

Ever since the fluoridation program was launched, the *Journal of the American Water Works Association* has carried articles and letters testifying to the difficulties and the hazards of fluoridation. A census of fluoridation published in the August 1953 *Journal* revealed the prevalence of corrosive damage to the fluoridation equipment and the mounting complaints of engineers all over the country that "the chemical flow is too free to permit accurate control."

In Schenectady, N. Y., the fluoridation equipment failed repeatedly. Valves became clogged and pumps stopped. As a result, in April of 1955, two years after the equipment was installed, fluoridation had actually been in operation for a period of only about 14 weeks. Alarmed by this fiasco, the Schenectady Taxpayers Association tried vainly to stop the program on the ground that it violated the Food and Drug Law.

In Morristown, N. J., which fluoridated its water in 1950, it was discovered, four years later, that the water coming from the taps in the Morristown hospital contained only 0.26 part per million of fluorine, while other outlets in the city varied from 0.44 part per million to none at all. This discovery was made by Dr. Reuben Feltman, who had been analyzing specimens of blood and placentas obtained through the cooperation of pathologists and obstetricians in the hospital.

Dr. Feltman's discovery, coupled with the Morristown water engineer's acknowledgment that he had been having continuous trouble with the fluoridating equipment, resulted in the scrapping of a survey of tooth decay among Morristown school children. The survey had been designed by the state health department to demonstrate the "success" of the fluoridation program. Instead, in May 1956 Morristown stopped fluoridating its water supply.

Pittsburgh, Pa., began fluoridating its water supply in December of 1951. Seven months later the water engineers were obliged to acknowledge that they hadn't yet been able to make the system function. More than enough fluoride had been dumped into the filtration plant, but not enough was coming out of the taps, and the engineers were rightly alarmed lest some of the trapped fluoride escape suddenly and release a dangerous excess into the drinking water.

Many of the towns and cities that have abandoned fluoridation have done so following the discovery that pipe and valve corrosion had made the fluoridation completely unreliable. In Northampton, Massachusetts, fluoridation was abandoned and the fluoridation equipment junked after it was found to be heavily corroded and clogged. Williamstown, Massachusetts, abandoned the program when the fluoridation equipment became unusable only two months after its installation.

Trouble with fluoridating equipment has been reported in many other cities, such as San Francisco, California; Sheridan, Wyoming; Coeur D'Alene, Idaho, and Martinez, California.

The chemical composition of ground water varies widely. Hence, it is not surprising that the addition of various forms of fluoride should give widely varying results.

No confidence can be placed in the statements made by local health authorities that the one-part-per-million level of fluoridation is being satisfactorily maintained. There is no such thing as a reliable standard test of the fluorine content of water.* At least a dozen procedures are being used currently and few of

---

* This was made abundantly clear at the 1956 conference of the American Water Works Association which heard reports of the inaccuracy and unreliability of the equipment used in fluoridation control.

them yield comparable results, the variations ranging over 100 percent. But even if accurate tests and reliable fluoridating equipment were available, the question, "One part per million of what?" would still have to be asked, and there is no way of answering it. A water distribution system is an environmental entity which may embody chemical deposits accumulated over a period of fifty years, depending upon the mineral and acid characteristics of the raw water. Fluorine can and does combine with other elements to form salts which vary widely in solubility and toxicity.

"Drop Out"

Equally unanswerable is the even more frightening problem of "drop out"—the accumulation, at critical points in the distributive system, of heavy deposits of highly toxic fluoride salts. The water engineer doesn't know where those deposits may occur and there is no way in which he can be sure that they will not suddenly be released in a quantity sufficient to push the fluoride dosage of the water consumer far above the threshold of tolerance. "Drop out," it must be remembered, is a cumulative phenomenon; a drop out or disappearance from the system of 0.1 part per million a day (which happens to be the smallest measurable quantity) could easily result, in the case of a large water system, in an accumulation within one year of several hundred pounds of toxic deposit.

The potential damage done to water drinkers by the drop out of added fluoride is likely to be slow and insidious; to industrial users it can be rapid and dramatic, as shown by the experience of the Meadow Brook Soft Water Laundry in North Andover, Massachusetts. The town fluoridated its water supply in 1953, and soon afterward, the laundry began to have trouble; often the entire laundry load would have a brown cast to it. To ascertain the cause of the trouble, the laundry spent thousands of dollars and enlisted the help of highly qualified consulting engineers. They found soft rust deposits nearly an inch thick in the laundry's hot water tank. Filters lined with baked enamel were covered with a deposit which, when removed, revealed that corrosion had removed the enamel and penetrated the steel. The intake pipe connecting with the town's water main clogged, leaked, and when removed was found to be corroded to paper thinness. What had happened was that fluoride had softened the heavy rust that had collected on the inside of the town's water mains over the years. As it freed itself it was carried along with the water and used by the people of North Andover—with consequences still to be determined by public-health officials who continue to deny that fluoridation presents problems to the water engineer.

At least one of these officials has even gone so far as to use his control of water system specifications and contracts as a means of pressuring water plant operating engineers into endorsing the program. In March of 1956, a selected list of New Jersey water engineers got a letter from a minor official in the state health department whose duties included that of passing on all plans and specifications for water works, chiefly water treatment plants, as to their adequacy under Health Department rules and regulations, and the qualifications of water plant operators to function as such. This official wrote:

> Fluoridation of public water supplies has been established as the greatest single contribution toward the promotion and protection of the public health in the water works business since the advent of chlorination . . . Fluoridation has not been accepted extensively in New Jersey . . . Today, however, we have reached the point where all the old bugaboos, all the old seemingly convincing arguments and all the excuses for opposing or postponing fluoridation have been dissipated. Even now there are some who could, if they would, advance the fluoridation program in this state but who prefer to take cover in the solace of passing the responsibility on to others . . . I need your help. Your reply

to this letter telling me how you feel about fluoridation today would be very helpful to me. I want to hear from you no matter what you think . . . *Your silence will not help.* If you disagree, your reply will not be publicized in any way; to the contrary I shall use your reply in opposition *for my information* and then destroy the letter." [Emphasis added]

A copy of this letter was forwarded to the writer by a water engineer who recalled uneasily the remarkable success enjoyed by a New Jersey manufacturer of chlorinators. For twenty-five years—until convicted in a federal court of violating the anti-trust laws—this manufacturer supplied more than 95 percent of the chlorinators in the entire country, despite the fact that its machines were matched by equipment of equal or greater merit produced by competitors. The same manufacturer now is a leader in the promotion of the fluoridation program and the sale of fluoridation equipment.

"As a public works engineer," wrote my correspondent, who is one of the recognized leaders of his profession, "made disgustingly familiar with all the variations of subsidized public officials, it has always been my belief that the monopoly enjoyed by this manufacturer was made possible by the venality of public officials in positions such as filled by the writer of this letter; this is the first time in the history of the department when any such pressure has taken this form of communication and I am wondering if commercial interests are not back of it. . . . I would dearly like to tear it [the letter] apart in a letter to ———— [the writer's superior officer] but to do so would subject my office to untold future difficulties in having our plans for water works approved by this same official."

The suspicions and apprehensions of this engineer may or may not have been well founded; the point is that the public health official in question was well aware that such apprehensions were and are shared by many public works engineers whose plans and specifications must run the gauntlet of his bureau.

Water department officials whose duties are those of management and operation are, of course, less subject to pressure, although they, too, are dependent upon approval of their qualifications by an examination of the State Health Department before their licenses can be issued.

In reply to the health department's demand that he stand up and be counted for or against fluoridation, Richard E. Bonyun, General Superintendent and Chief Engineer of the Passaic Valley Water Commission, replied as follows:

> This subject was first brought to the attention of the Passaic Valley Water Commissioners in 1949 and my opinion and recommendations were requested. After serious consideration I recommended that the fluoridation of the public water supply under their control be not undertaken, and set forth the reasons for my recommendation.
>
> Since that time I have attended many meetings on the subject, read many articles (pro and con) with an open mind and still hold to my original opinion and personal views thereon . . . I do not consider it the proper function of a public water supply to treat or reduce the incidence of any particular disease which is not communicable or which is not a public health hazard to all of the consuming public. Dental caries can be treated or its incidence minimized by the personal action of those individuals who seek or desire such treatment.
>
> I disagree wholeheartedly with those who contend that fluoridation is not different in principle from chlorination and that the reason for the almost universal acceptance of the latter can be used as an argument in favor of the former. As I see it, the chlorination of a public water supply is to kill bacteria which may be present in the water and which would be harmful to the entire population served and would, therefore, constitute a public health hazard. Fluoridation of a public water supply is for the purpose of adding to the water an element which is not naturally present and which might be of some benefit to some people in the community and the addition of which would be, if not harmful, of no benefit to others. The absence of fluorides in a public water supply does not constitute a public health hazard.

It is not necessary for you to keep this letter in strict confidence since I have on many occasions openly expressed my views herein contained.

Without question Mr. Bonyun's views are those of the majority of American water engineers. Many of them go considerably farther. At a conference of the Maine Water Utilities Association, Portland, Maine, in February of 1956, B. C. Nesin, Director of Laboratories of the Department of Water Supply, Gas and Electricity of New York City, said:

There can be no question of the hazards involved in fluoridation and any idea of maintaining a public health flirtation with it is nothing more than so much macabre, pseudo-scientific sophistry. The whole concept of fluoridation is a perversion of the hard-earned experience acquired in the development of safe water supply practice . . .

The continued promotion of water supply fluoridation in face of mounting adverse evidence and criticism requires some evaluation. It seems that the proponents hit upon an idea years ago which appealed to them, and which they felt was sound. As their claims of safety were progressively discredited, rather than acknowledge this, they persisted in condoning such evidence. At the same time they were lending their prestige to such equivocation. Certainly the proponents of fluoridation are not intent upon poisoning or harming anyone. However, the dilemma of prestige is a very difficult matter to resolve.

The proponents have tried to demonstrate various factors of safety which are patently naïve. They speak of factors of safety of 2, or 8, etc. with little comprehension of the meaning of this term in water supply practice. A factor of safety of 2 or 8 on their terms is no factor of safety at all. It has been customary to consider a minimal factor of safety of not less than 10 for substances which may be admitted to water supplies. This would mean that ten times the amount of the proposed substance when present in the water supply would be definitely without harm to human or beast. It is obvious from the knowledge of fluoride toxicity that such a factor of safety cannot be established when fluoride is added to the public water supply at the level recommended by the proponents of fluoridation. In view of the fact that the range of water consumption may vary over a ratio of 20 to 1, the insistence upon a factor of safety of 10 is exceedingly moderate.

It must be concluded that the fluoridation of public water supplies is a hazardous procedure. People are bound to get hurt. It remains to find out how many and when. I do not believe the water supply fraternity is interested in demonstrating this with wholesale experimentation on populations.

Mr. Nesin is the author of a half dozen studies of the scientific background of fluoridation, including the most comprehensive review of the literature of fluoride poisoning as related to water supplies that has yet been published. Of him, even more than of most water engineers, it must be acknowledged that he knows his subject. Moreover, since he and his colleagues are not dependent upon Public Health Service grants, there would seem to be no way by which they can be brain-washed into conformity with the official fluoridation gospel.

Future historians may record this as a most fortunate circumstance.

Alternatives to Fluoridation

IF the public health service is genuinely interested in reducing the incidence of tooth decay, not only among children but in the total population, there exists a safe and effective alternative to water fluoridation.

It is an educational program designed to reduce the consumption, especially by children, of sugar and sugar-containing foods and beverages.

Such a program would not be the least experimental, nor would it involve the slightest risk to either children or adults. Sugar rationing in two wars has proved that the less sugar, the less tooth decay. This finding has been confirmed by many controlled studies, including those of Dr. Clive M. McCay at Cornell. Dr. McCay's rat studies have shown that the sugar and phosphoric acid content of soft drinks tends to destroy tooth enamel and increase the incidence of caries among both children and adults. He has urged a tax on soft drinks, the proceeds to be applied to the free distribution of milk—which helps to build good teeth and bones—in school lunches.

Even if the Public Health Service were to limit such an alternative program to "local level" campaigns by school authorities against the excessive consumption of soft drinks and candy bars, past experience has shown that it could count on a substantial measure of success in reducing tooth decay as well as an appreciable improvement of the nutritional and health status of both children and adults.

If, however, the Public Health Service desired to obtain such debatable benefits in the reduction or postponement of caries as may be obtained by the administration of fluoride in controlled dosage to children under twelve, then the alternative "pill program" suggested by the New York City Health Department is clearly preferable to the fluoridation of the water supply. It is relatively safe, far cheaper, and embodies no elements of compulsion. The City Council of Newark, New Jersey, adopted such a "pill program."

Twenty years ago, some of the leading proponents of the fluoridation thesis envisaged topical application of fluorides, the free distribution of fluoride pills, or the incorporation of pharmaceutical grade fluorides in milk or salt as the preferred methods of fluorine application. The subsequent insistence of the Public Health Service on municipal water fluoridation or nothing is inexplicable in terms of normal public health policy and practice; in fact the reasons given for the rejection of these alternative methods are so manifestly baseless as to seem disingenuous.

In 1939, C. J. Cox suggested that in addition to water supplies ". . . other media such as bottled water, and milk supply and fluorine-containing medicals are feasible; and that the means of control of fluorine in the whole dietary of children should be undertaken." [1] Seven years later, in discussing the dental caries findings of the U. S. Public Health Service research group, Francis A. Arnold said:

These results permit the following assumptions in regard to the action of fluorides on dental caries: First, it is not essential for fluorides to be continuously present in the diet for more than the first eight years of life in order that caries be inhibited. Secondly, the inhibitory action of fluorine may be dependent on the presence of optimal quantities in the diet during the formative period of the teeth, presumably increasing the fluoride content of the enamel and the dentin.

On the basis of studies on daily water consumption of children, McClure has calculated that the average child has a daily intake of about one milligram of fluorine when using a fluoride drinking water containing one part per million of fluorine. Thus, by supplementing the daily diet of a child using a fluoride-free water supply with one milligram of fluorine, we might expect a beneficial effect on the dental caries experience of that child. . . . During the first two years, the child's drinking water and also the water used in preparing any special formula, can be made to contain one part per million of fluorine. This may be done by adding the desired amount of a solution of NaF of proper concentration or by the use of sodium fluoride tablets of known weight. For example, one cubic centimeter of a solution of sodium fluorine which contains 2.21 milligrams sodium fluoride when added to one liter of water will result in drinking water containing one part per million of fluorine. After the child has reached the age where the source of his drinking water varies, i.e., sometimes at home and sometimes away from home, his diet may be supplemented by the addition of 2.21 milligrams sodium fluoride added daily to a glass of drinking water, fruit juice or milk.[2]

The fluoridation thesis which Dr. Arnold was then upholding has remained unchanged so far as the Public Health Service is concerned. Today, as in 1946, it is "easy and simple," as Dr. Arnold then stated, to get one part per million of added fluorine into a child's diet by the use of standard fluorine tablets administered by the parents.* How did it happen, then, that in 1956 the U. S. Public Health Service was obstinately opposing

* Similar programs, such as the voluntary administration of vitamin A to young children, have prevented rickets in the United States and elsewhere.

the easy, simple, democratic and relatively safe "pill program" that was its method of choice a decade earlier?

In her report to the Mayor of New York on fluoridation for New York City, Health Commissioner Leona Baumgartner even went so far as to allege that the fluoridation of water supplies, with its inevitable variations in fluoride intake of over 500 percent, represented a safer and more reliable means of controlling fluorine dosage than the daily consumption of a tablet containing one milligram of fluorine, dissolved in a glass of water. A similar hardihood appears in Dr. Baumgartner's analysis of comparative costs. The pill program, she estimates, would cost at least $1.00 per hundred, making the cost per person protected about $3.65 a year. Actually, the unit cost of pharmaceutical grade sodium fluoride tablets purchased by the city from the same suppliers as those used by the municipal hospitals in their purchase of other pharmaceuticals would be *not $1.00 per hundred, but 25 cents per thousand*. Errors of this magnitude can hardly be achieved unintentionally.

The true basis of comparison is set forth in B. C. Nesin's report to the New York City's Department of Water Supply, Gas and Electricity on "Various Means of Providing Fluoride Intake for Prevention of Dental Caries in Children." Mr. Nesin's estimate is that it would cost New York City about $110,000 a year to make a carefully administered "pill program" available to the city's entire child population of approximately 1,500,000 in the age group under twelve. This is slightly more than one tenth of the million dollars a year that fluoridation of the municipal water system would cost, not counting added expense from probable increases in the market price of fluorides and fluoridating machinery and even more probable increases in the cost of maintaining fluoride-clogged and corroded water lines.

A comparison of the relative advantages of three methods of fluoride administration (municipal fluoridation, home supply of fluoride water and tablets containing fluorides) is given in Table 6, which appears on page 215. It is based on the tabulation of Dietz[3] as revised by Nesin in the report of the New York City Department of Water Supply, Gas and Electricity already referred to. Note that in this comparison the tablet program is superior in all respects except ease of administration and applicability to urban children. Significantly, the Swiss, who thus far have avoided any experimentation with municipal water fluoridation, have for some years been conducting controlled experiments with tablet administration on a voluntary basis.

A number of other proposals for providing supplementary fluoride intake have been made. Milk, sugar, flour and salt have all been suggested as carriers for fluorides, the purchaser to be given his choice of the fluoridated and fluorine-free forms of these staples. All of these methods, like the present provision of iodized and iodine-free salt, are preferable to municipal water fluoridation in that they are voluntary as well as less hazardous. None of them, however, is as inexpensive or as controllable as the use of fluoride tablets.

An obvious advantage of the pill program is that it does not subject allergic and kidney deficient children and adults to a mass treatment that is admittedly contraindicated for such individuals. Parents are not obliged to give their children fluoride pills unless they and their physicians think it desirable. If they do, and adverse effects result from this controlled treatment, it can be promptly discontinued. That something of this sort would happen is indicated by Dr. Reuben Feltman's preliminary report,[4] showing that of 1100 pregnant women and children given daily tablet doses of one part per million of fluorine, eleven experienced adverse effects.

The adoption of a pill program by a great or even a small city would provide a relatively huge sample from which the medical fraternity might expect to learn much that is not now known concerning the effects and symptomatology of fluoride poisoning. Judging from what is now known, however, it would seem probable that the ultimate result of such an experiment would be the abandonment of the fluoridation thesis, the prohibition of any further public health flirtation with the most lethal of the halogens, and a salutary shift toward saner methods of dealing with tooth decay.

TABLE 6

(In a discussion of the efficiency of fluoridation comparing tablets, bottled water prepared with tablets, and water supply fluoridation Dietz (11) has formulated a comparative decigrade chart showing the advantages and disadvantages of the various methods. In his first totalization, tablets were credited with 7 A's, 3 B's; bottled water, 7 B's, 3 C's; and water supply, 3 A's, 7 C's. In his scoring A is most favorable, B is intermediate, and C is least favorable. The following tabulation is a revision of Dietz's Table 2 in accordance with the findings discussed in the present report.)

Decigrade Comparison of Advantages and Disadvantages of Various Methods of Providing Fluoride to Children.

(Based upon Dietz, Table 2, (11), revised)

A comparative decigrade chart showing advantages and disadvantages of various methods. These attributes are weighted from A—most favorable to C—least favorable. Each column contains an arbitrarily and mutually exclusive "ABC" classification.

	Municipal Fluoridation	Home Supply Fluoride Water	Tablets Containing Fluoride
Ease of administration	A	C	B
Precision in dosage	C	B	A
Applicability to rural children	C	B	A
Applicability to urban children	A	C	B
Reported effectiveness	C (50-70%)	B (60-70%)*	A (75%)
Effect on primary teeth	C	B	A
Effect on permanent teeth	C	B	A
Avoidance of fluoridated water for adults or other uses	C	B	A
Exclusive control by dental, medical and related professions ..	C	B	A
Cost	C	B	A
Total	2 A's 8 C's	8 B's 2 C's	8 A's 2 B's

* Theoretical.

(The revision in the above tabulation concerns mainly the item of cost.)

Revolt of the Human

Test Animals

EVEN today, over a decade after fluoridation was started in the pilot-plant cities, and six years after the program was formally launched by the Public Health Service, it is probable that nine out of ten of the 28,000,000 Americans living in the fluoridated cities don't realize that they are drinking water to which one part per million of fluoride has been added.

As citizens and taxpayers, their approval was clearly necessary before they could be made the subjects of an experiment involving an admitted and more or less calculated risk to their health. No such consent would have been obtained if the program had been honestly presented to Congress. Hence the "local level" approval is one that the Public Health Service devised to "engineer the consent" of its human test animals.

Actually, their consent was not even "engineered," in many cases; it was simply by-passed. The health department, with the tacit consent of some mayors and/or city councils, bought the fluoridation equipment and put the program into operation weeks or months before it was announced in the newspapers.

In other cases, the public was deliberately deceived by a false announcement that the program had been initiated, thus giving some of the human test animals a chance to register fear of fluoride poisoning and even psychosomatic complaints. This enabled the Public Health Service, after fluoridation was actually in operation, to cite these imaginary illnesses as proof that all subsequent cases of fluoride intoxication must be confined to neurotics, no matter how clearly their complaints were supported by clinical evidence. Indeed, there are strong indications that some of these complaints were "planted" by proponents of fluoridation.

A necessarily incomplete list of the regional and local organizations that comprise the fluoridation resistance movement will to be found in Appendix 4. Since January 1955 the movement has been provided with a monthly national journal.*

Although adherents of the unorthodox healing cults have been active in organizing many of these groups, they are by this time greatly outnumbered by orthodox members of the American Medical Association and the American Dental Association, who have taken the time to appraise critically the controversial proponent literature; also by miscellaneous laymen of every race, creed and color who find common cause in their unwillingness to subject themselves and their families to a risk which originally was considered calculated but turned out to be incalculable.

If the human test animals are given sufficient advance warning they are usually able to prevent the local health officer, the

* *The National Fluoridation News,* a nonprofit publication edited by Mrs. George L. Waldbott, and published at 2930 West Grand Boulevard, Detroit 2, Mich. Mrs. Waldbott, wife of Dr. George L. Waldbott, one of the authors of this book, is assisted by a group of advisory editors consisting of distinguished members of the medical, dental, chemical and legal professions.

mayor and/or members of the city council from railroading the community into the fluoridation experiment. They first organize a broadly based emergency committee which includes qualified professionals—doctors, dentists, chemists, engineers, lawyers, etc. This committee demands postponement of any action regarding fluoridation pending the investigation and report of an advisory committee which must include qualified representatives of the opposition to the program, even if it is necessary to import professionals from outside the community. Regardless of the recommendations of this committee, opponents of the program can insist that the issue be submitted to a popular referendum; if necessary, they can go to court to prevent arbitrary action by the city council or the health authorities.

Half the battle is won by preventing a coup by proponents of the program. Past experience shows that where a referendum election is held, fluoridation is defeated nine times out of ten. When the proponents win it is usually because the opposition permits itself to be divided along sectarian lines, because it fails to make adequate use of the scientific evidence against the program, such as is assembled in this book, or because, in a one-newspaper town, it is denied the democratic right of free and fair public discussion of the issue. In the latter case the opposition has successfully taken to the advertising columns of the newspaper, using the "$1,000 Reward" device that helped to repeal fluoridation in Charlottesville, Virginia, and elsewhere, in defeating the initiation of the program or in bringing about its abandonment.

Such advertisements, which summarize the damning evidence that the program is dangerous, offer a reward to anyone who can refute it. This involves no risk whatever to opponents of the program. Well aware that this evidence is massive and irrefutable, proponents of the program have to date made few attempts to collect the rewards.

To break through a press censorship, where it exists, it is also important to make maximum use of local and network radio and television time. Since the air media are by law operated to serve the "public interest and necessity" those not wishing to serve as test animals can properly demand time on the air to answer the lavish and unscrupulous propaganda of the United States Public Health Service experimenters. Where this demand is refused, opponents of the program have succeeded by appealing to the Federal Communications Commission.

If, despite all efforts, the proponents win, either by action of the City Council or in a popular referendum, opponents usually regard this as only the first round. Recourse to the courts will often win a postponement of the program, pending the consideration of new evidence by the City Council. As this book is being written, a number of cities which have adopted fluoridation have delayed putting the program into effect because of sharp increases in the price of fluorides. In others, suspension of the program has been brought about either by the failure of the fluoridation equipment, or by increasing evidence of fluoride poisoning, affecting both people and domestic animals, in the fluoridated cities.

It would seem that the tide turned in favor of the fluoridation resistance movement in 1952, when fluoridation was defeated in Seattle. Since then, the curve of adoption has declined and the number of communities abandoning the program has steadily increased. The score, as this book goes to press, is as follows:

In some 400 fluoridated communities, approximately 28,000,000 human test animals are either swallowing fluoridated water drawn from the taps, or are evading the experiment by buying fluorine-free bottled water; the number of the latter is steadily increasing as evidence of fluoride poisoning mounts in the cities that have been fluoridated for three or more years.

More than balancing this record are the 660 cities, with a population of about 40,000,000, that have thus far either rejected fluoridation or have abandoned it after trials ranging in duration from a few months to four years.

At least four cities—Sacramento, California; Worcester, Massachusetts; Dover-Foxcroft, Maine, and Vancouver, British Columbia, Canada, have rejected the program three times running. In five communities—Salem, Oregon; Syracuse, New York; Needham, Massachusetts; Fairfield, Califorina, and Albany, Oregon— the proposal to fluoridate has been twice defeated.

Some 75 cities, with several others probable at this writing, have abandoned fluoridation after trials of varying periods, and have sold or junked their fluoridating equipment. A list of these cities, as of September 1, 1956, is given in Appendix 2.

At the national level, the fluoridation resistance movement has brought about two Congressional Inquiries: by the House Select Committee to Investigate the use of Chemicals in Foods and Cosmetics in January–March of 1952, and by the House Committee on Interstate and Foreign Commerce in May of 1954. The published hearings of these two committees are among the most valuable sources of evidence against the fluoridation program.

The House Select Committee on Chemicals in Foods was composed of the following seven members: James J. Delaney, New York, Chairman; Thomas G. Abernethy, Mississippi; E.H. Hedrick, West Virginia; Paul C. Jones, Missouri; A. L. Miller, Nebraska; Gordon L. McDonough, California; and Walt Horan, Washington. Congressmen Hedrick and Miller are medical doctors, and Dr. Miller is a former Health Commissioner of Nebraska. Vincent A. Kleinfeld, one of the most able and experienced food and drug lawyers in Washington, served as chief counsel of the committee, which heard a total of eighteen testimonies, including eleven proponents and seven opponents of the fluoridation program.

It is significant that both Dr. Miller, who had helped to introduce fluoridation in the District of Columbia, and Mr. Kleinfeld, whose past professional associations might have been expected to incline him favorably toward the U. S. Public Health Service, were convinced by their examinations of the witnesses that fluoridation was still an experiment, so laden with potential dangers that America should go very slowly about extending it. Even more significant is the fact that the committee members, who differed violently on every other issue they considered, voted unanimously to sign the Committee's "Go Slow" recommendations. The report reads:

> The area of controversy concerning the fluoridation of water arises over the question whether a sufficient amount of investigation and study has been completed to justify a

recommendation of universal application of this procedure at this time. . . . The view of the minority group is that . . . it is not known with any degree of certainty exactly what subtle physiological effects may ensue and that a number of important questions remain unanswered.

Proponents of fluoridation rely heavily . . . upon the vital statistics of communities which have had natural fluorides in their drinking water for many years, to prove that inhabitants of such areas are not afflicted with any different or more serious illnesses than persons from nonfluoride areas. . . . This type of study is contrasted with a clinical study in which the observations remain related to the particular individual. . . .

It was the opinion of some of the witnesses that vital statistics could not be relied upon to determine whether the physical conditions of particular persons, such as those afflicted with a kidney ailment, would or would not be made worse by the ingestion of fluoridated water.

None of the pilot experiments has been completed. It is estimated that a minimum of ten years is required to assess the advantages and disadvantages, if any, of these programs. At least one of these studies is designed as a 15-year study. In none of them is the adult or old-age population being studied to determine what physiological effects fluoridated water will have on these groups.

The Committee is not concerned with the term "mass medication." The important problem is not whether fluoridation is, or is not mass medication, but whether it contains any hazards to any portion of the population. Nevertheless, since the question was raised at the hearings, the committee wishes to point out that the fluoridation program does constitute medication, and medication without parallel in the history of medicine. Water is consumed by every person in a community, regardless of his age, physical condition, or possible personal reactions. It is essential, therefore, that all the facts concerning fluoridation be disseminated, and an opportunity given to people of each community to decide for themselves whether they desire to assume, at this time, the calculated risk inherent in the program. . . . The committee believes that if communities are to mistake in reaching a decision . . . it is better to err on the side of caution.

Impressive as was this sober warning, it was not enough for Dr. Miller who, perhaps more than any other member of the committee, was equipped by training and experience to appraise the evidence presented at the hearings. In a personal statement supplementing the committee's report, Dr. Miller wrote:

> In my opinion, the United States Public Health Service has been premature in urging universal use of fluorides in water. They have gone beyond the scope of their duties or what was expected of them by Congress and the people. . . . The Public Health Service should concern itself with good public health measures and the prevention of disease. If it goes into the propaganda field, it will lose its effectiveness and the confidence of the public.
>
> In reading the testimony, we do find that the very people of the United States Public Health Service, who now so earnestly urge the use of fluorides in drinking water, were, as late as 1950, according to their published papers, saying: "The evaluation of the effects of fluorides in drinking water has not been established and must wait until the experiments, now in progress, are completed."
>
> I am convinced that many of the groups who now endorse fluorides in water are merely parroting each other's opinions. They have done no original research work themselves. . . . In my opinion, there is no urgency about the matter.

Two years after the release of the Delaney Committee's "Go Slow" report, the fluoridation resistance movement staged a desperate effort to scotch the fluoridation program at its source, in Washington. A bill (HR 2341) was introduced in the 83rd Congress by Representative Roy W. Wier of Minnesota. It would have prohibited any agency of government, whether federal, state or local, from treating any public water supply with any fluoride compound.

Even the bill's sponsors probably realized that it would not be passed. Since the U. S. Public Health Service had not attempted to introduce fluoridation nationally, the program could scarcely be stopped by the direct intervention of Congress. If fluoridation was to be defeated, it would have to be fought town by town and city by city in hundreds of "local level" engagements.

The bill had great strategic value, however, because it provided a national forum in which the opponents of fluoridation could and did prove, both that fluoridation was still an experiment, four years after its national application had been urged by the U. S. Public Health Service, and that the "calculated" risk to the human test animals was greater than had been supposed.

In 1952, proponents of the program had admitted to the Delaney Committee that no experiments had been conducted to test the safety of fluoridation for kidney deficient children or, especially, for kidney deficient men over sixty, about half of whom suffer from prostate enlargement which often reduces kidney function to as little as 5 percent. ("Let 'em drink bottled water," suggested Dr. F. F. Heyroth of the Kettering Institute in Cincinnati, Ohio.)

Two years later the same proponents told the Wolverton Committee, not only that they still had no experimental answers to this question, but that no such experiments were contemplated. (They are still neither in progress nor contemplated by the U. S. Public Health Service, so far as is known, although every qualified internist recognizes the special suspectibility of kidney deficient subjects to fluoride poisoning.)

In 1952, little was said at the hearings of the Delaney Committee about the promotional enormities committed by the proponents of fluoridation: their suppression and manipulation of evidence, their dissemination of half truths and outright falsifications, and their slander of opponents.

But, in 1954, the opponents of the program read into the record of the Wolverton Committee's hearings damning excerpts from the secret minutes of the Fourth Annual Conference of State Dental Directors with the Public Health Service and the Children's Bureau, proving that behind closed doors, the proponents of the program plotted and urged precisely such promotional methods.

In the end, the great controversy over fluoridation will be decided not so much by political action on a local or a national level, as by accumulated scientific evidence. Already this evidence is beginning to make medical and other scientific groups reverse their former stands.

For instance, the Texas Medical Society, in April, 1956, unanimously refused to endorse fluoridation and decided not to consider the question for another five years. The Wayne County Medical Society in Detroit, after a committee had studied some of the evidence on fluoride poisoning, rescinded its previous endorsement of fluoridation, July 6, 1956, and is taking a neutral stand on the subject. The New Orleans Board of Health opposes fluoridation. The Board of Health in Spartanburg, South Carolina, after a careful study of the problem, has openly warned against fluoridation. The Health Commissioner of Phoenix, Arizona, has also recently rejected an effort to obtain fluoridation in his town.

A thirty-three-member citizens' advisory committee appointed by Mayor T. T. Tabor of Madison, New Jersey, after carefully studying the scientific evidence, came out strongly against fluoridation of water supplies. Its reason: the permanent benefit to teeth has not been proven; there are great doubts regarding its safety; the dose cannot be controlled when a drug is added to drinking water; dental caries is not a contagious disease and, therefore, should be dealt with on an individual basis; dispensing fluorides by physicians and dentists individually is a safer and less expensive method. Fluoridation is an invasion of the constitutional rights in the absence of demonstrated necessity to protect the health of the community, there is inadequate research on fluoridation; it is uneconomical.

In 1952, only a handful of scientists outside the U. S. Public Health Service officialdom had equipped themselves to appraise ⋯lation or, indeed, given the program any serious attention.

By 1954, there were scores and by now there are hundreds of physicians, dentists, biochemists, and other health workers all across the country who have read the literature of fluorine poisoning, compared it with the official statements of the U. S. Public Health Service and registered their shock and amazement at what they found.

It is on these men whom the fluoridation resistance movement must pin its faith. Not all of them can be intimidated and silenced. It is they—and the evidence they are gathering of what fluoridation has already done to the captive human test animals on whom it has been imposed—who may be counted upon to end the American fluoridation experiment before it becomes a national disaster.

APPENDICES

APPENDIX 1

How the Public Health Service Answers Questioners

BY JAMES RORTY

PROFESSIONAL and lay persons who have had no prior acquaintance with the methods used to promote the fluoridation program assume quite naturally that questions addressed to the Public Health Service will be answered frankly and accurately. The following exchange of letters, between the writer and Dr. John W. Knutson, Assistant Surgeon General and Chief Dental Officer of the Public Health Service, shows that this assumption is unwarranted.—J.R.

July 8, 1956

Dr. John W. Knutson, Assistant Surgeon General
Chief Dental Officer, PHS
Public Health Service,
Washington, D. C.

Dear Dr. Knutson:

For use in a book in preparation on the fluoridation of municipal water supplies, can you supply me with some or all of the following data?

1. What is the present number of communities that have adopted fluoridation? What is their population? If available, please provide me with a detailed list of cities, towns and water systems in which fluoridation is in operation, with dates when the program was adopted.

2. What communities have adopted fluoridation and subsequently abandoned the program? For what reasons?

3. What communities have adopted fluoridation by popular referendum? Without popular referendum?

4. In what communities has fluoridation been proposed and rejected? By popular referendum? Without referendum?

5. Dr. Reuben Feltman, 211 Main Avenue, Passaic, N. J., has recently made public the preliminary findings of his study of a thousand pregnant women and young children to whom fluoride tablets were administered at a dosage of 1 ppm. His preliminary findings indicate that approximately 0.7 of his subjects reacted so adversely to the treatment that it had to be discontinued. How do you regard these findings? Dr. Feltman's studies were originally financed by a Public Health Service grant, which was subsequently discontinued. Why was it discontinued?

6. Dr. George L. Waldbott's paper on "Chronic Fluorine Intoxication from Drinking Water" (*Int. Arch. Allergy* 7, 70-74, 1955) has been followed by studies, soon to be published, of some 52 cases of incipient fluorine intoxication from drinking water. In her report to the Mayor of New York City on fluoridation, Dr. Leona Baumgartner discounts Dr. Waldbott's reports on the ground that in her view the "rules of scientific investigation" were not observed by Dr. Waldbott in his observation of these cases. Has the Public Health Service undertaken any investigation of these and similar cases now being reported from the fluoridated cities? If not, does the Public Health Service feel no obligation to conduct studies, by accepted scientific methods, that will establish whether or not these and similar cases, all of

which exhibit the recognized syndrome of fluorine poisoning, are in fact caused by fluorine poisoning?

7. In view of the increasing reports of fluorine poisoning in the fluoridated cities, and in view of recent laboratory studies (Wallace-Durbin, William Ramsyer at Cornell, and others) which tend to destroy the premises on which the fluoridation program is based, it has been urged by qualified and responsible physicians and other health workers that the fluoridation program be discontinued. I am in fact informed that the desirability of such a discontinuance has been discussed by the Public Health Service. Is this information correct?

8. Recently a number of communities have postponed or discontinued fluoridation because of the scarcity and high prices of fluorides. Can you inform me concerning these price rises and their explanation?

9. Recently, water engineers have reported "fall-out" of the fluorides introduced into water systems, with resulting inability to maintain a constant 1 ppm dosage and risk of sudden release of excessive amounts of fluorides into the systems. There have also been reports of corrosion of transmission lines and the failure of fluoridation equipment. Is your department aware of these reports and how does it appraise them? Leading water engineers, including Commissioner Ford of New York City, say it is impossible to guarantee the maintenance of a safe dosage. Is it not true that unless water engineers can guarantee the maintenance of the recommended dosage, within a margin of safety recognized as adequate, then, regardless of all other considerations, the program is not safe?

10. Commissioner Ford states that it would cost the City less than 25 cents for a thousand days to distribute fluoride tablets free through health stations for parents to administer to children, so that the cost of such an alternative program would be less than one fifth of the cost of a fluoridated water program. Is this an accurate estimate in your opinion? What, if any, are your objections to the "pill" program?

You will agree, I am sure, that in view of the importance of the issue, I am obligated to ask these questions, so that, as a responsible journalist, I may avoid any possible misrepresentation of the Public Health Service. I shall feel equally obligated to print your answers in full in the book which will shortly be delivered to the publisher, so that there can be no question of quoting out of context.

Sincerely yours,
James Rorty

August 9, 1956

Mr. James Rorty
Flatbrookville
New Jersey

Dear Mr. Rorty:

I am sorry that an answer to your letter of July 8 has been delayed by my absence from this office on official business and by the time required to compile the information you requested. Here are answers to the questions submitted in your letter:

1-4. As of July 27, 1956, according to the best information available to the Public Health Service, a total of 1,390 communities including some 27.5 million people had adopted the practice of controlled fluoridation of public water supplies to reduce the incidence of dental caries. I regret that we are unable to furnish a list of cities, towns and water supplies of the type you wish to obtain. However, I enclose 6 statistical tables which present data answering in large part the questions raised under your first four headings.

5. Dr. Feltman's statements are indeed contradictory to the Public Health Service recommendation that the adjustment of the fluoride content of public water supplies is a safe, effective, and economical procedure for the partial prevention of tooth decay.

Dr. Feltman received his Public Health Service Research grants from the National Institute of Dental Research, during the period August 1950–August 1955. His original research application proposed "to determine the efficacy (in preventing caries) of the addition of measured doses of fluoride salts to pregnant women and to children up to and through the age of eight years." It was considered a worthy research project and still is.

Dr. Feltman's request for financial support for this study was reviewed from time to time by members of the Dental Study Section and by the National Advisory Council on Dental Research. The Study Section and the Council are made up of non-governmental scientists and representatives of the public, serving in an advisory capacity to the Public Health Service. The most recent action by these groups was to terminate financial support for his project, because in their opinion, Dr. Feltman had not reached his objective and was not likely to do so.

One of the problems encountered by Dr. Feltman in conducting this study, according to one of his progress reports to the National Institute of Dental Research, was that after the study had progressed for a considerable period of time it was found that many of his "control" patients had been receiving prenatal medication, chiefly various types of calcium tablets, which contained appreciable quantities of fluoride. This meant that many members of his "control" group were not receiving appreciably different levels of fluorides than the members of his "experimental" group who had been fed fluoride tablets. Any interpretation of the results of this project to determine the effects of fluoride tablets on pregnant women would therefore be open to very serious question.

Two publications attributed to the research conducted under these grants are "Pre-natal and post-natal ingestion of fluoride," J. Dent. Med. 6:48-52 (1951), and "The fluoride content of placental tissue as related to fluoride content of drinking water," Science, 115 (1952). These publications obviously stem from the early years of Public Health Service support of Dr. Feltman's research. Investigators receiving financial assistance from the Public Health Service are requested to submit a final report within 30 days after completion of the research project. To date, Dr. Feltman has not submitted this report.

Of the publications and progress reports submitted by Dr. Feltman to the National Institute of Dental Research, none mention any kind of ill effects to the persons taking the fluoride pills. If Dr. Feltman has such evidence, he has not cited it in any of his material submitted in his request for grants. In point of fact, there are no data based on careful scientific research to indicate that waterborne fluoride ingestion at the levels used for dental decay control has any general ill effects.

6. To our knowledge, no scientific evidence to support Dr. George Waldbott's views on water fluoridation has been published in any medical journal in this country. Whenever his claims have been considered by competent committees or groups

studying the subject of water fluoridation, no basis for his conclusions have been found. For example, an inquiry among the physicians in Grand Rapids, Michigan, where the water has been fluoridated for more than twelve years, revealed that the conditions described by Dr. Waldbott were non-existent.

This observation is supported also by the statement made in November, 1955, by Dr. Hildebrand, Health Officer of Sheboygan, Wisconsin, where fluoridation was started in 1946: "Sheboygan's 48 physicians last year issued a statement that they had noticed no adverse effect on any of their patients that could be attributed to fluoridation. But they had noticed a marked decrease in tooth decay in children."

The Wayne County (Michigan) Medical Society, of which Dr. Waldbott is a member, issued the following statement on February 6, 1956: "At the request of Dr. Waldbott, the Committee reconsidered the question of water fluoridation. Since in the opinion of the Committee, Dr. Waldbott did not submit sufficient evidence to substantiate his charge that water fluoridation is a health hazard, it was recommended that the Wayne County Medical Society reaffirm its previous action endorsing fluoridation subject to certain specific controls outlined by the Detroit Department of Health."

The Florida State Board of Health heard testimony from Dr. Waldbott in an extensive consideration of its water fluoridation policy. After these deliberations, the State Board of Health's previous position endorsing water fluoridation was reaffirmed.

Incidentally, Dr. Baumgartner's assessment of Dr. Waldbott's reports is confirmed by the findings of a German scientist, Dr. Hornung, who came to this country last year to study water fluoridation. Dr. Hornung discussed the subject at some length with Dr. Waldbott and obtained a copy of his survey form. Upon returning to Germany, Dr. Hornung conducted a survey in a German community which had a chlorinated but low fluoride drinking water supply so he substituted the word chlorine for the word fluorine in the survey form. The results of his survey are of particular interest since the incidence of complaints of the conditions Dr. Waldbott attributes to fluorine was higher when associated with the water chlorination than with water fluoridation.

7. Scientists of the Public Health Service, universities, and other research centers are aware of the effects of *excessive*

amounts of fluoride on human life. The natural occurrence of fluorides in public water supplies serving a considerable part of our population has afforded an excellent natural laboratory in which to study these effects. Studies of individuals who had drunk water containing *excessive* amounts of fluoride all their life found that no significant physiological or functional effects resulted except mottled tooth enamel. In mortality studies, no statistically significant difference was found between the death rates in fluoride and non-fluoride cities for all causes of death. The same was true for death rates due specifically to heart disease, cancer, intracranial lesions, nephritis, or cirrhosis of the liver—conditions whose possible relation to fluoridation has been suggested.

On the other hand, the effectiveness of the controlled addition of an optimum amount of fluorides to public water supplies has been demonstrated in independently conducted studies in Grand Rapids, Michigan; Newburgh, New York; Brantford, Ontario; Marshall, Texas; and other places. All of these studies found that tooth decay was markedly reduced as a result of fluoridation.

The Public Health Service, after many years of careful study and observation, including a review of independent investigations, concluded that the controlled fluoridation of public water supplies is a safe, effective, and economical procedure for the partial prevention of tooth decay. In keeping with its legal and professional obligations to make known its findings on public health matters, the Public Health Service has continuously reported its findings on fluoridation to health agencies throughout the Nation. No change in this policy has ever been considered.

The major organizations concerned with the health of the nation, such as the American Dental Association, the American Medical Association, the American Public Health Association, the American Association for the Advancement of Science, the National Research Council, and many others, have endorsed fluoridation, like the Public Health Service, only after careful review of all the scientific evidence.

Inasmuch as Dr. Ramsyer of Cornell University has not yet published the results of his studies on the effect of fluoride supplements in the diet of rats, I am not familiar with his findings. Nevertheless, experience with such studies suggests that it would be well for you to make a careful check on the amount of the fluoride supplement. It is not unlikely that the basic diet of the rats contained 10 to 15 ppm of fluorine and that the drinking water contained an additional 10 to 15 ppm. If this be the case then the results are associated with 20 to 30 times the optimum fluoride concentration. Furthermore, it would represent another of the many instances in which the opponents of fluoridation rest their case on the erroneous assumption that the proponents of fluoridation do not recognize and acknowledge the undesirable effects of *excessive* fluorides.

8. The Public Health Service is now gathering information concerning the shortage of fluoride chemicals which caused the temporary discontinuance of fluoridation recently in a few communities. As of August 1, 1956, reports from 34 States and Territories indicated that, during the latter part of 1955 and the early part of 1956, some 23 communities stopped fluoridation for periods ranging from a few days to four months solely because of a shortage of fluoride chemicals. In addition, 2 communities are known to have delayed fluoridation somewhat because of this shortage.

Our information indicates that the shortage of fluoride chemicals was precipitated by a strike in the Florida phosphate fields during the summer of 1955. The resulting shortage of supply was aggravated by curtailed production elsewhere in the United States and by a lack of fluorides available for import. The most important factor contributing to the shortage was increased industrial use of silicofluorides here and abroad for making steel and various enameled products. The shortage of fluoride chemicals has now been substantially alleviated. All but 4 of the 23 communities mentioned above have now resumed fluoridation.

There has been some rise in the price of fluorides over the years, but it appears to be commensurate with increases in the cost of other commodities. For example, the sodium fluoride purchased for Grand Rapids, Michigan, in 1947 averaged $10.90 CWT, and in 1955, $14.30 CWT—an increase of 31 percent. Between 1947 and 1955, the wholesale price index for inorganic chemicals and allied products rose from 93.1 to 132.0—an increase of 42 percent. The data for sodium fluoride purchases [are] believed to be typical of the increased cost of other fluoride compounds.

9. We are not aware of any reliably reported "fallout" or "buildup" of fluorides in the water systems of the nearly 1400

communities now supplementing the fluoride content of their water. Our experience in over ten years of operating the Grand Rapids fluoridation project indicates that we maintain the optimum concentration of 1 part per million with a variance of much less than 1/10 part per million. This performance can be achieved in any water system where competent operators follow reasonably careful procedures.

Moreover, there are no corroborated reports of transmission line erosion or failure of transmission lines in fluoridated systems that may be attributed to fluoridation. There is no evidence, indeed, even to suggest that a stable concentration of fluoride cannot be maintained in all parts of a water distribution system at all times, including such large systems as, for example, those serving Chicago and Philadelphia.

10. The use of fluoride-bearing tablets for the widespread control of dental caries has never been considered seriously in this country. To our knowledge, the only U. S. community which has attempted to solve its dental health problems in this way has been Newark, New Jersey. In Newark, the City Council recently directed the Health Department to make tablets containing 0.5 milligrams fluoride available to those who might wish to use them. The tablets are obtainable at no cost from the Health Department upon presentation of a prescription from a physician or a dentist. Dr. A. H. Haskin, City Health Officer, has informed us that at the end of the first six weeks only three prescriptions had been presented.

A limited number of Swiss communities distribute tablets through the school system. A program of this type has the obvious defect of not reaching the child of pre-school age—a most critical period for tooth formation. In addition, the distribution of fluoride bearing tablets on a community-wide basis is not a practical public health procedure because of the virtual impossibility of assuring proper use of the tablets over long periods of time.

Tablets containing 1/2 milligram fluoride may be purchased for 65¢ per thousand. Although Commissioner Ford assumes that these tablets are to be used by all children, he neglects to estimate the overhead costs of achieving cooperation from all the citizens of the community for a program of this kind. This would be highly expensive, if it could in fact be accomplished at all.

We appreciate the opportunity to furnish factual information with respect to fluoridation of public water supplies. If we can be of further assistance, please call upon us.

> Sincerely yours,
> John W. Knutson
> Assistant General Surgeon
> Chief Dental Officer, PHS

Enclosure

A REVIEW AND ANALYSIS OF
DR. KNUTSON'S ANSWERS

1-4. As Dr. Knutson acknowledges, the Public Health Service's statistical tables provide only incomplete answers to the questions asked. Hence the authors of this book have been obliged to rely on the facts and figures compiled by Mrs. Arthur R. Robinson of Seattle, Washington, which are given in Appendix 2. They show merely that the information provided by Dr. Knutson was both incomplete and somewhat outdated.

5. Dr. Knutson's answers to this question are so wholly unjust that in all fairness they demand correction. The actual history of Dr. Feltman's project is as follows: After starting his research with his own funds, Dr. Feltman obtained, in 1950, a Public Health Service grant, conditioned upon the assurance given by Dr. Feltman and by the Passaic General Hospital that the study would be continued for a minimum of ten years, and that Dr. Feltman would report the facts as he found them. He states that the reasons given for discontinuing Public Health Service support of the project are not based on fact. Dr. Feltman reported the presence of fluoride in calcium tablets customarily prescribed for pregnant women as soon as it was determined. Obviously, the same factor affected both Dr. Feltman's subjects and his controls. Dr. Feltman points out that if Dr. Knutson's objection is valid, then the reports from anywhere in the country, including the Public Health Service's studies in Newburgh, Grand Rapids, and Brantford, Ontario, are "open to serious question," since the same pharmaceuticals are prescribed everywhere, with no notation of fluoride content on the label. Regarding his failure to submit a terminal report, Dr. Feltman points out that his project has years to go yet, that he published

two papers in 1956 based on his studies, and that on the completion of these studies he has every intention of furnishing the Public Health Service with a full report. Dr. Feltman further observes that Dr. Knutson is in error in stating that "there are no data based on careful scientific research to indicate that waterborne fluoride ingestion at the levels used for dental decay control has any general ill effects." Actually, there are cases being treated in the East and Midwest for fluoride intoxication from drinking water.

6. Neither the Committee of the Wayne County Medical Society to which Dr. Knutson referred nor Dr. Baumgartner nor the Florida State Board of Health has had access to, much less reviewed, Dr. Waldbott's case reports. After a special committee of the Wayne County Medical Society, appointed to examine Dr. Waldbott's evidence on poisoning, had studied *some* of his cases, they recommended that the Council of the Society take a neutral stand. This was accepted by the Council on July 6, 1956. Dr. Knutson's office was promptly informed of this action.

Dr. Waldbott has letters from medical editors proving that the Public Health Service has been preventing publication of his poisoning reports in American medical journals. This does not, of course, discredit such reports when published abroad in scientific journals of high standing, as is the case with Dr. Waldbott's studies. Concerning the findings of Dr. Hornung, a health officer, not a physician, Dr. Waldbott points out that Dr. Hornung has acknowledged his complete ignorance of chronic incipient fluoride poisoning and that no competent clinician would consider his survey to be bona fide research. On the other hand, Dr. Waldbott's studies are not based on a survey but on personal observations.

7. Does Dr. Knutson consider an inquiry among Grand Rapids physicians, who admittedly have no knowledge of the disease, scientific evidence? Dr. Knutson must be aware that research scientists responsible to or employed by the Public Health Service (whose names I am pledged not to reveal) are disturbed by their own findings and by those of other scientists whose more recent studies have discredited the studies of McClure and others on which the fluoridation premise is based. Significantly, Dr. Knutson ignores my question as to whether or not these scientists have recommended discontinuance of the

program. Dr. Knutson's attempt to discredit in advance, and without seeing them, the findings of Dr. William Ramsyer is even more astonishing, since representatives of the Public Health Service were among the first to visit Cornell, examine Dr. Ramsyer's slides, and listen to the tape record of the doctoral thesis which describes his studies and reports his findings. As the Public Health Service, if not Dr. Knutson himself, must be well aware, the premises on which Dr. Knutson bases his attempt to discredit Dr. Ramsyer are purely imaginary. In summary, Dr. Ramsyer's experiments consisted in feeding albino rats sodium fluoride at 1, 5, and 10 ppm levels ad libitum in their drinking water. At the age of 520 days, corresponding to about 42 years in a human being, he killed 86 animals that had been drinking water fluoridated at the 1 ppm level. They had *more* tooth decay and *more* periodontal lesions than the controls. The 520-day-old rats that had been getting 1 ppm of fluoride also showed definite kidney lesions. *All* the 520-day-old animals showed some interstitial nephritis, and those that got the most fluoride showed the most severe nephritis. *All* the 520-day-old animals also showed periodontal lesions. Dr. Ramsyer's conclusion: that fluoride at 1 ppm does not prevent tooth decay but seems to increase periodontal disease during gestation and lactation periods and for the remainder of these lives.

8. Dr. Knutson's figures on the increased cost of fluorides will be read with amazement by water engineers and mayors who have been unable to buy fluorides at any such "average" prices.

9. Dr. Knutson's statement that the experience of Grand Rapids shows maintenance of the "optimum" concentration of 1 part per million with a variance of much less than 1/10 of a part per million is flatly contradicted by the facts of record. The actual figures for Grand Rapids during the month of January 1954 were published in the report on H.R. 2341, page 333, as furnished by William Leslie Harris, Superintendent of the Water Department, City of Grand Rapids. During this one month the fluoride content in the clear well varied from 1.02 to 1.19 ppm. In various outlets reported, it varied from 0.98 to 1.19 ppm. From various taps on the same day it varied from 1.07 to 1.19. From the same tap on different days it varied in one case from 1.03 to 1.14; in another from 0.98 to 1.14; in another from 1.01 to 1.19. From one tap, on successive days, it varied from 1.11 to 1.01 to 1.14. One wonders:

what are the sources of Dr. Knutson's statement, since he can scarcely be ignorant of the January 1954 report? Is it reasonable to assume that the engineers picked the worst month in ten years to report?

Dr. Knutson is, likewise, incorrect when he denies the existence of evidence of "fall-out" and erosion or failure of transmission lines in fluoridated water systems. The reader will find some of this evidence in Chapter 8; it is based on the reports of responsible water engineers, delivered at professional conferences, and much of it subsequently published.

10. I asked Dr. Knutson if New York City's Water Commissioner, Arthur Ford, was accurate in stating that fluoride tablets could be purchased for 25 cents per thousand. He evades the question by saying that such tablets "may be purchased for 65 cents per thousand." The fact, of course, is that fluoride tablets *can* be purchased at 25 cents per thousand, as Dr. Knutson must be quite aware. For other evaded facts on the alternative "pill program," see Chapter 9.

James Rorty

Communities Discarding

Artificial Fluoridation

The following cities, towns, and villages in the United States have discarded artificial fluoridation of public water supplies after test periods of varying durations. This tabulation was compiled as of September 1, 1956, by Mrs. Arthur R. Robinson, Seattle 5, Wash.

Martinez, Calif.
Rio Vista, Calif.
San Diego, Calif.
　Del Mar, Calif.
　La Jolla, Calif.
　Part of Coronado, Calif.
　San Diequito, Calif.
　Santa Fe, Calif.
Mount Dora, Fla.
Coeur D'Alene, Ida.

Lewiston Orchards, Ida.
St. Maries, Ida.
Geneseo, Ill.
Indianola, Ill.
Knoxville, Iowa
Wakeeney, Kan.
Minneapolis, Kan.
Franklin, Ky.
Port Sulphur, La.
St. Martinsville, La.

Bangor, Me.
Hudson, Mass.
Northampton, Mass.
Williamstown, Mass.
Bay City, Mich.
Grosse Pointe, Mich.
Ishpeming, Mich.
Saginaw, Mich.
Austin, Minn.
Faribault, Minn.
Bay Spring, Miss.
Polson, Mont.
Fort Belknap, Mont.
Beatrice, Neb.
Amsterdam, N. Y.
Fulton, N. Y.
Schenectady, N. Y.
Tuckahoe, N. Y.
Greensboro, N. C.
  Guilford College, N. C.
  Hamilton Lakes, N. C.
Gastonia, N. C.
Akron, O.
Jackson, O.
Greenville, S. C.
  Fountain Inn, S. C.
  Marietta, S. C.
  Mauldin, S. C.

Simpsonville, S. C.
Slater, S. C.
Travelers Rest, S. C.
Donaldson AF Base, S. C.
Tyler, Tex.
Wichita Falls, Tex.
Blackstone, Va.
Charlottesville, Va.
Kennewick, Wash.
Hinton, W. Va.
Princeton, W. Va.
New Martinsville, W. Va.
Bucholz, Wis.
Blooming Grove, Wis.
Delavan, Wis.
Elroy, Wis.
Gillet, Wis.
LaCrosse, Wis.
Markesan, Wis.
Platteville, Wis.
Prairie DuSac, Wis.
Rhinelander, Wis.
Stevens Point, Wis.
Westby, Wis.
Weyauwega, Wis.
Whispering Pines, Wis.
Sheridan, Wyo.

APPENDIX $\boxed{3}$

Fluoridation—The Unbelievable Blunder

BY K. K. PALUEV*

THE FIRST ERROR: PREMATURE PROMISES OF THE U. S. PUBLIC HEALTH SERVICE AND THE AMERICAN DENTAL ASSOCIATION

In the words of Dr. David M. Ast,† *et al.,* the Newburgh artificial fluoridation of public water was an experiment to determine

* Mr. Paluev, a Fellow of the American Institute of Electrical Engineers, is an experienced analyst of experimental data. He has been for several decades a research and development engineer for a large corporation and is the author of many technical papers, the holder of many patents, and the recipient of professional and civic awards. He has filed five bills on fluoridation with the Massachusetts Legislature and has testified in Congressional hearings on matters pertaining to fluoridation. He also testified in January 1956 before the New York City Committee on Health and Education. He has presented his fluoridation findings to the first Inter-professional Conference on Fluoridation (March 1956).

† Director of the Newburgh, New York, experiment.

the "efficacy and safety of this caries prophylactic measure." They also state that three-fourths of all caries is found among permanent molars. (Report Number I—June 1950.)

In the words of Dr. Bruce D. Forsyth, Assistant Surgeon General, Chief Dental Officer, U. S. Public Health Service, the experiments "were set for a minimum of ten years." (HR 74, page 1508.)

The Newburgh experiment was initiated in May 1945, the Grand Rapids experiment in January 1945.

Until 1948–1949 the U. S. Public Health Service opposed artificial fluoridation and favored direct or topical application of fluoride compounds to teeth.

In 1949 Dr. John W. Knutson, Assistant Surgeon General of the U. S., published an article explaining the best method of topical application. Concurrently, a U. S. Public Health Service pamphlet appeared, under the signature of Oscar R. Ewing (Dr. Knutson's boss), declaring: "Direct application of certain fluorine preparations to the teeth is the *only* method of proven effectiveness."

However, in June 1950, Dr. Leonard Scheele, the U. S. Surgeon General, declared before the Congressional Committee that the U. S. Public Health Service gave an "unqualified endorsement" to water fluoridation (HR 74, page 1500). A little later, Dr. Knutson, in promoting water fluoridation, demanded, "Why are we quibbling, delaying, pigeon-holing, in the face of exhaustive research and overwhelming proof?" He promised, further, ". . . two-thirds fewer cavities and extractions," ". . . straighter, stronger, better looking teeth" for generations raised on fluoridated waters and, further, that ". . . these benefits are not temporary, they last a lifetime." (Paper read before the Massachusetts Dental Convention, January 17, 1952.)

Dr. Ast and other leading official proponents insist that only persons born *after* fluoridation was introduced can provide significant data.

Children born in 1945 in Newburgh or Grand Rapids *did not have a single permanent tooth even erupted by 1950* and, therefore, could not provide any evidence in support of the stand taken by the U. S. Public Health Service and endorsed by The American Dental Association the same year. Even by 1955, at the end of 10 years of experiments, the average duration of usage of permanent teeth by the 10-year-olds was only three years; of the normal set of 28 teeth, they had only 14 erupted one or more years and only half of the eight molars erupted. However, as explained here, by 1955 they provided sufficient evidence to prove the inability of fluoridated water to reduce DMF (decayed, missing, filled teeth).

THE SECOND ERROR: DELAY IS TAKEN FOR REDUCTION

My analysis of the official experimental evidence of the effect on tooth decay of fluoride dissolved in public waters in Newburgh, New York, and Grand Rapids convinced me that *no measurable reduction in decay was found there* as compared with conditions prevailing in these cities before inauguration of fluoridation. The difference in decay found before and after ten years of fluoridation is simply in the age in which a given level of decay (the number of decayed, missing, and filled teeth) has been found. The official data indicate that any given level of decay present in children living before fluoridation was found among fluoridated children, whether of the same age or slightly older (but not more than 2.3 years older).

In other words, when individuals born after fluoridation of public waters become *young adults*, they will have, in these cities, the *same amount of accumulated dental trouble as their non-fluoridated predecessors have had. They will not have 60% less,* as every member of the New York City Board of Health and millions of others were led to believe by the U. S. Public Health Service and The American Dental Association announcements.

Even among 8-year-olds born in *Newburgh and Grand Rapids after fluoridation* was initiated, the dental decay is very severe. For example, out of four permanent molars erupted *two or three years* earlier, the following decay was detected:

> One DMF or more in 3 out of every 4 children
> Two DMF or more in 1 out of every 3 children
> Three DMF or more in 1 out of every 10 children.

Thus, no less than *half of the molars were DMF among one-third of the children* by the age of eight. Obviously, Dr. Knutson's promise has failed.

THE THIRD ERROR

Another fallacy of the method is in expressing "reductions" in percentages. This is illustrated by the following example, where the rate of increase in DMF per year and the accumulated number of DMF in the two groups of children are identical, except that Group B lags one year behind Group A. Yet, by the official promoters' methods "reduction up to 100% with the average of 54% is demonstrated," to use the familiar words of the U. S. Public Health Service and The American Dental Association announcements.

AVERAGE DMF PER CHILD

AGE	6	7	8	9	10	
Group A	0.5	2.0	3.5	5.0	6.5	
Group B	0.0	0.5	2.0	3.5	5.0	
Difference	0.5	1.5	1.5	1.5	1.5	
"Reduction" %	100	75	43	30	23	54% average

THE FOURTH ERROR: AVERAGING "REDUCTIONS"

The percentual "reductions" in the table above decline radically in five years.

Not even an extremely inexperienced analyst would average these reductions and thereby disguise the decline. Yet, such averages as "60% reduction" are driven into the public mind through TV, radio, newspapers, magazines, and even books by the U. S. Public Health Service, The American Dental Association, and other well-meaning but misguided associations and individuals.

THE FIFTH ERROR

A prophylactic helpful only to a very mild decay is of little value. However, the official method used for the evaluation of possible beneficial effects of fluoride disguises such characteristics, because the number of DMF contains the entire range of decayed teeth from the slightly afflicted to the completely lost. It is quite likely that, among 6- to 10-year-old children, slightly decayed teeth account for a large portion of this number. If fluoride only *delays* detection of decay, such an effect would obviously affect the slightly decayed first, that is, the greatest number. This would markedly reduce the number of DMF reported, giving fallacious impressions of a marked prophylactic effect.

Dr. Ast *et al.*, in Report I, stated that their study ". . . shows that artificially fluoridated water had the greatest prophylactic effect during the period of this study on the teeth least often attacked by caries."

APPENDIX 4

Organizations Comprising the Fluoridation-

Resistance Movement, October 31, 1956

National Committee Against Fluoridation, 1311 G St. NW, Washington 5, D. C.

State Groups:

Pure Water Association of America Inc., California Committee, P. O. Box 600, Palo Alto, Calif.

Tennessee Pure Water Association, McQueen Farm, Loudon, Tenn.

Florida Pure Water Association, 321 South Massachusetts Ave., Lakeland, Fla.

Nebraska Citizens Against Fluoridation, Lincoln and Omaha, Neb.

Health Freedom League of Arkansas, Box 1071, Fort Smith, Ark.

Fluoridation Educational Society of the Carolinas, 900 South Duke St., Durham, N. C.

New York State Committee of Pure Water Association, Beacon, N. Y.

Pennsylvania Citizens' Committee Against Fluoridation, Lancaster, Pa.

Washington State Anti-Fluoridation League, 5217 East 43rd St., Seattle, Wash.

New Jersey Citizens Against Fluoridation, Glen Ridge, Westfield, and Trenton, N. J.

Salt Lake Citizens Against Fluoridation, Salt Lake City, Utah.

Others

Citizens' Medical Ref. Bureau, Setauket, N. Y.

Etowah County Pure Water Association, Box 267, Gadsden, Ala.

Citizens' Pure Water Committee, 112 Lewis St., San Diego, Calif.

Greenville, S. C., Citizens Against Fluoridation, Apt. 4B, McDaniel Heights Apartments, Greenville, N. C.

Portland Citizens' Committee Against Fluoridation, Portland, Ore.

Citizens' Committee Against Fluoridation, P. O. Box 7041, Atlanta, Ga.

Citizens' Committee Against Fluoridation, 6632 South Lowe Ave., Chicago 21, Ill.

Dickinson County Anti-Fluoridation Council, Box 334, Iron Mountain, Mich.

Fluoridation Research Committee (Against Fluoridation), Saginaw, Mich.

Citizens Against Fluoridation, Cincinnati, Ohio.

Citizens Against Fluoridation, 546 South Prairie, Okmulgee, Okla.

Prevention magazine, Emmaus, Pa.

Wichita Falls, Texas, Citizens Against Fluoridation, Wichita Falls, Tex.

LaCrosse Citizens' Committee Against Fluoridation, Box 713, LaCrosse, Wis.

Americanism Bulletin, Box 141, Galva, Ill.

Tecumseh Anti-Fluoridation Committee, P. O. Box 621, Tecumseh, Mich.

Butte Citizens' Pure Water Committee, 2810 Phillips St., Butte, Mont.

Greater New York Committee Opposed to Fluoridation, 175 5th Ave., New York 10, N. Y.

Pomona Anti-Fluoridation Association, P. O. Box 375, Pomona, Calif.

Lee Foundation, Milwaukee, Wis.

NOTES

CHAPTER 2

1. *Hearings Before the House Select Committee to Investigate the Use of Chemicals in Foods and Cosmetics,* House of Representatives, 82nd Congress, Second Session. Part 3, p. 1619. 2. H. E. Wirth, "Engineering Control and Maintenance of Artificial Fluoridation of Communal Water Supplies," *Fluoridation of Public Water Supplies, A Symposium,* University of Washington, April 27, 1951. 3. News article, the *Pittsburgh Press,* August 2, 1953. Photo copy available from: National Committee Against Fluoridation, Inc., 1311 G St., N. W., Room 601, Washington 5, D. C. 4. R. Feltman, "Letter to the Editor," *J.N.J. Dent. Soc.* 25:37, September 1954. 5. H. T. Dean, F. S. McKay, and E. Elvove, "Mottled Enamel Survey of Bauxite, Arkansas, Ten Years After a Change in the Common Water Supply," *Pub. Health Rep.* 53:1736-1748, September 30, 1938. Also H. T. Dean, "Domestic Water and Dental Caries," *Pub. Health Rep.* 56:378, February 28, 1941. 6. "News of Dentistry: Public Health," *J.A.D.A.* 50:484, April 1955. 7. "Water Fluoridation: Report of the Committee of the St. Louis Medical Society." *J. Missouri Med. Assn.* 51:126-142, February 1954. 8. H. T. Dean, Philip Jay, F. A. Arnold, Jr., and E. Elvove, "Domestic Water and Dental Caries II," *Pub. Health Rep.* 56:762-792, April 11, 1941. 9. A.D.A. *Newsletter,* 8:4, April 15, 1955. 10. F. J. McClure, "Nondental Physiological Effects of Trace Quantities of Fluorine," *Dental Caries and Fluorine, A Symposium,* F. R. Moulton, ed., A.A.A.S., Washington, D. C., 1946, p. 74-92. 11. F. J. McClure, H. M. Mitchell, T. S. Hamilton and C. A. Kinsen, "Balances of Fluorine Ingested from Various Sources in Food and Water by Five Young Men," *J. Indust. Hyg. & Toxicol.* 27:159-170, June 1945. 12. F. J. McClure, "Ingestion of Fluoride and Dental Caries," *Am. J. Dis. Child.* 66:362-369, 1943. 13. Report of the Ad Hoc Committee of the National Research Council. 14. F. J. McClure, "Fluoride Domestic Waters and Systemic Effects, II., Fluorine Content of Urine in Relation to Fluorine in Drinking Water." *Pub. Health Rep.* 59:1575-1590, December 8, 1944. 15. F. J. McClure, "Fluorine and Other Trace Elements in Nutrition," *A.M.A. Handbook of Nutrition,* 2nd ed., London, Lewis, 1951, p. 146. 16. McClure, Mitchell, Hamilton, and Kinsen, *op. cit.,* p. 162. 17. "Caries Control Workshop," University of Michigan, *J. Dent. Res.* 27: 267-272, p. 276. 18. McClure, "Nondental Physiological Effects of Trace Quantities of Fluorine," p. 80. 19. Patricia Wallace-Durbin, "The Metabolism of Fluorine in the Rat Using F^{18} As a Tracer," *J. Dent. Res.* 33:797, December 1954. 20. "Health Department Answers Questions on Fluoridation," Washington State Department of Health, *The Bellevue American,* April 7, 1955. 21. F. J. McClure,

"Fluoride Domestic Waters and Systemic Effects I., Relation to Bone-fracture Experience," *Pub. Health Rep.* 59:1543-1558, December 1, 1944. **22.** John W. Knutson, "The Case for Water Fluoridation," *New England Journal of Medicine* 246:737-743, May 8, 1952. **23.** E. R. Hammarlund, "Why All the Delay on Fluoridation?" *J. Am. Pharmaceutical Ass'n.* 16:22-26, January 1955, p. 23. **24.** I. N. Hill, D. E. Jelinek and J. R. Blayney, "Evanston Dental Caries Study, Preliminary Study of Distribution of Fluorine in Communal Water Supplies in the U. S.," *J. Dent. Res.* 28:398-414, August 1949. **25.** P. E. Mooler and S. V. Gudjonsson, "Massive Fluorosis of Bones and Ligaments," *Acta radiol.* 13:269-294, 1932. **26.** Kaj Roholm, *Fluorine Intoxication: A Clinical-hygienic Study,* Lewis, London, 1937. **27.** H. E. Shortt, G. R. McRobert, T. W. Barnard and A. S. M. Nayar, "Endemic Fluorosis in the Madras Presidency," *Indian J. M. Res.* 25:553-568, October 1937. **28.** C. G. Pandit, T. N. S. Raghavachari, R. Subba and V. Krishnamurti, "Endemic Fluorosis in South India," *Indian J. M. Res.,* October 1940. **29.** E. Speder, "L'Ostéopetrose de la Fluorose Phosphatique de l'Afrique du Nord," *Bull. et Mém. Soc. de Radio. Méd. de France* 24:200-207, 1938 (the abstract in the *Yearbook of Radiology,* 1936, p. 79, is from another article in *J. de Radiol. et d'électrol.* 20:1-10, January 1936). **30.** T. Ockerse, "Endemic Fluorosis in the Pretoria District," *South African M. J.* 15:261-266, 1941. **31.** Pandit, Raghavachari, Subba and Krishnamurti, *op. cit.,* p. 538. **32.** E. J. Largent, W. Machle and I. J. Ferneau, Jr., "Fluoride Ingestion and Bone Changes in Experimental Animals," *J. Indust. Hyg. & Toxicol.* 25:396-408, November 1943. **33.** A. W. Pierce, "Chronic Fluorine Intoxication in Domestic Animals," *Nutrition Abstr. & Rev.,* University of Adelaide, Adelaide, Australia, 9:14, p. 1939. **34.** Bartolucci, quoted by Roholm in *Fluorine Intoxication.* **35.** L. L. Silva, E. Chapedi and E. A. Pedace, "Fluorosis y Tuberculosis," *La Semana Medica,* 24:1413-1434, June 13, 1940. **36.** J. R. Lemmon, "Enamel of Teeth in Children," *Texas State J. M.* 30:332-336, September 1934. (Also quoted by H. T. Dean, "Chronic Endemic Dental Fluorosis," *J.A.M.A.* 107:1269-1273, October 17, 1936.) **37.** Report by Commission on Chronic Illness, *Chronic Illness News Letter,* April 1954. Commission on Chronic Illness, 615 North Wolff St., Baltimore 5, Md. **38.** Theodore R. Van Dellen, syndicated column, "How to Keep Well," *Seattle Times,* April 24, 1955. **39.** J. F. Linsman and C. A. McMurray, "Fluoride Osteosclerosis from Drinking Water," *Radiology* 40:474-484, June 1943. See also *Radiology* 41:497, November 1943, for correction of misprint. **40.** *Hearings Before the House Select Committee,* pp. 1655-1956. **41.** Largent, Machle, Ferneau, *op. cit.* **42.** *Hearings Before the House Select Committee,* p. 1673. **43.** McClure, "Nondental Physiological Effects of Trace Quantities of Fluorine." **44.** Thomas L.

Hagan, Morton Pasternack and Grace C. Scholz, "Waterborne Fluorides and Mortality," *Pub. Health Rep.* 69:450-454, May 1954. **45.** Iowa State Department of Health, Division of Public Health Engineering, "Fluoride in Public Water Supplies of Iowa," *Iowa Public Health Bulletin*, Des Moines, The Department, 1950. **46.** *Hearings Before the Committee on Interstate and Foreign Commerce of the House of Representatives*, 83rd Congress, Second Session, on H. R. 2341, A Bill to Protect the Public Health from the Dangers of Fluoridation of Water, p. 377. **47.** *Hearings Before the House Select Com.*, pp. 1664-66. **48.** J. Gershon-Cohen and J. F. McClendon, "Roentgen Studies of Osteoporosis II: The Inhibitive Effect of Dietary Phosphate Fertilizer on Dental Caries and Skeletal Decalcification in the Rat," *Am. J. Roentgenol.* 72:247-249, August 1954. **49.** *Hearings Before the House Select Committee*, pp. 1530-1532; 1644-1666. **50.** *Hearings Before the Committee on Interstate and Foreign Commerce*, pp. 307-308. **51.** *Ibid.*, p. 258. **52.** Report by Commission on Chronic Illness. **53.** *Hearings Before the House Select Committee*, pp. 371-372. **54.** E. R. Zimmerman, N. C. Leone and F. A. Arnold, Jr., "Oral Aspects and Excessive Fluorides in a Water Supply," *J.A.D.A.* 50:272-277, March 1955. **55.** N. C. Leone, F. A. Arnold, Jr., E. R. Zimmerman, P. B. Geiser and J. A. Liebermann, "Review of the Bartlett-Cameron Survey; A Ten Year Fluoride Study," *J.A.D.A.* 50:277-281, March 1955. **56.** Texas State Department of Health, *Fluoride Concentrations in Public Water Supplies in Texas, Based on Analyses from 1937-1952*, Austin, The Department, 1952. **57.** R. W. Sundstrom, W. W. Hastings and W. L. Broadhurst, "Public Water Supplies in Eastern Texas," *Geological Survey Water Supply Paper*, No. 1047, Washington, D. C., U. S. G.P.O., 1948. **58.** *Hearings Before the Committee on Interstate and Foreign Commerce*, table on p. 333. **59.** J. F. McClure, "Review of Fluorine and Its Physiological Effects," *Physiol. Rev.* 13:295-297, July 1933. **60.** McClure, "Nondental Physiological Effects of Trace Quantities of Fluorine," p. 89. **61.** Leone, Arnold, Zimmermann, Geiser and Liebermann, *op. cit.* **62.** McClure, "Review of Fluorine and Its Physiological Effects," p. 295. **63.** Leone, Arnold, Zimmermann, Geiser and Liebermann, *op. cit.* **64.** Leo Spira, "Mottled Nails, An Early Sign of Fluorosis." *J. Hyg.* 43:69, 1943. **65.** Leo Spira, "The Aetiology of Otosclerosis," *J. Laryng. & Otol.* 43:151-157, April 1943. **66.** McClure, "Review of Fluorine and Its Physiological Effects," p. 289. **67.** McClure, "Nondental Physiological Effects of Trace Quantities of Fluorine," p. 89. **68.** McClure, "Review of Fluorine and Its Physiological Effects." **69.** Hans Borei, "Inhibition of Cellular Oxidation by Fluoride," *Arkiv. for Kemi, Mineralogioch Geologi*, utgivet av K. Svenska Veterskapsakademien, Band 20 A. No. 8. Almqvist & Wiksells Boktryckeri, A. B. Stockholm (also London, Lewis), 1945, pp. 9, 10, and 50. **70.** J. F. Fazekas and H. E. Himwich, "The Significance of a Pathway of Carbohydrate Breakdown Not Involving Glycolysis," *J. Biol. Chem.* 139:971-972, June 1941. See also: J. F. Fazekas, F. A. D. Alexander, and H. E. Himwich, "Tolerance of Newborn to Anoxia," *Am. J. Physiol.* 134:281, 1941; and H. E. Himwich, A. Birnstein, H. C. Herrlick, A. Chessler and J. F. Fazekas, "Mechanism for Maintenance of Life in Newborn During Anoxia," *Am. J. Physiol.* 135:387, 1942.

CHAPTER 3

1. F. S. McKay, "Mottled Enamel: Early History and Unique Features," *Symposium on Fluorine and Dental Health,* American Association for the Advancement of Science, Washington, D. C., 1942, p. 1. **2.** F. S. McKay, "An Investigation of Mottled Teeth," *Dental Cosmos* 58:477-484, May; 627-644, June; 781-792, July; 894-904, August 1916. **3.** J. M. Eager, "Chiaie Teeth," *Dental Cosmos* 43:300-301, March 1902. **4.** H. A. Fynn, "Some Remarks on Defects in Enamel of Children of Colorado Springs," *Dental Items of Interest* 32:31-34, 1910. Also, *Brit. J. Dent. Sci.* 53:215-218, 1910. **5.** O. W. Holmes, "The Claims of Dentistry," Commencement Address, *Missouri Dent. J.* 4:161-179, May 1872. **6.** F. Maury, *Treatise on the Dental Art, Founded on Actual Experience.* Translated from the German by J. B. Savier, Philadelphia, Lea & Blanchard, 1843, pp. 73-75. **7.** John Hunter, *A Practical Treatise on the Diseases of the Teeth,* Part II, London, American Society of Dental Surgeons, 1771, p. 2. Reprint in *American Library of Dental Science,* New York, 1839. **8.** Ph. Fr. Blandin, *Anatomy of the Dental System, Human and Comparative.* Translated from the French by Robert Arthur. Baltimore, American Society of Dental Surgeons, 1845. **9.** G. V. Black, *A Work on Operative Dentistry* (chapter by McKay), Chicago, Medico-Dental Publishing Co., 1936, 7th ed., p. 221. **10.** G. V. Black, *A Work on Operative Dentistry,* Chicago, Medico-Dental Publishing Co., 1920, vol. 1, 4th ed., p. 43. **11.** L. P. Meredith, *The Teeth and How to Save Them,* London, William Tegg and Co., 1878, 2nd ed., pp. 152-153. **12.** I. Schour and M. C. Smith, "Experimental Dental Fluorosis," *Fluorine and Dental Health,* A.A.A.S., Washington, D. C., 1942, p. 47. **13.** C. Dillon, "Pathological Significance of Mottled Teeth," *Dent. Pract.* 3:366-375, August 1953. Also C. Dillon, "Biochemistry of Fluoride," *Dent. Digest* 59:486-490, November 1953. **14.** R. F. Soggnaes, "A Condition Suggestive of Threshold Dental Fluorosis Observed in Tristan da Cunha," *J. Dent. Res.* 20:303-313, August 1941. **15.** H. S. Fleming and V. S. Greenfield, "Changes in the Teeth and Jaws of Neonatal Webster Mice after the Administration of NaF and CaF_2

to the Female Parent During Gestation," *J. Dent. Res.* 33:780-788, December 1954. **16.** P. Wallace-Durbin, "The Metabolism of Fluorine in the Rat Using F^{18} as a Tracer," *J. Dent. Res.* 33:789-800, December 1954. **17.** A. L. Russell and E. Elvove, "Domestic Water and Dental Caries, VII: A Study of the Fluoride-dental Caries Relationship in an Adult Population," *Pub. Health Rep.* 66:1389-1401, October 26, 1951, p. 1398. **18.** E. R. Zimmermann, N. C. Leone and F. A. Arnold, "Oral Aspects of Excessive Fluorides in a Water Supply," *J.A.D.A.* 50:272-277, March 1955, p. 274. **19.** Meredith, *op. cit.* **20.** G. V. Black and F. S. McKay, "Mottled Teeth," *Dental Cosmos,* 58:129-156, February 1916. **21.** C. H. Boissevain, "Presence of Fluorine in Water Supply of Colorado and Its Relation to Occurrence of Mottled Enamel," *Colorado Med.* 30:142-148, April 1933, p. 147. **22.** M. C. Smith and H. V. Smith, "Observations on Durability of Mottled Teeth," *Am. J. Pub. Health* 30:1050-1052, September 1940. **23.** *Proceedings,* Fourth Annual Conference of State Dental Directors with the PHS and the Children's Bureau, Federal Security Building, Washington, D. C., June 6-8, 1951. **24.** APHA Conference Report, "No Evidence of Pathoses from Fluoride Ingestion," *Pub. Health Rep.* 68:223, February 1953. **25.** Boissevain, *op. cit.* **26.** J. G. Frisch, "Alteration of Dental Enamel Structure by 'Natural' and 'Added' Fluoride in the Human," *J. Wisc. State Dent. Soc.* 24:127-130, July 1948. **27.** M. Massler and I. Schour, "Relation of Endemic Dental Fluorosis to Malnutrition," *J.A.D.A.* 44:156-165, February 1952. **28.** O. E. Hoffman, Testimony under Cross-examination, In Re: Kaul *vs.* City of Chehalis, in the Superior Court of the State of Washington in and for the County of Lewis, October 1, 1952. **29.** *Hearings Before the House Select Committee to Investigate the Use of Chemicals in Foods and Cosmetics,* House of Representatives, 82nd Congress, Washington, D. C., Government Printing Office, 1952, Part 3, p. 1650. **30.** C. Dillon, "Fluorine and Dental Caries," *Dent. Pract.* 3:79-86, November 1952. C. Dillon, "Method of Determining Calcium-precipitating Fluorine Salts in Drinking Water and the Causation of Mottling," *Dent. Pract.* 3:101-104, December 1952. **31.** G. J. Cox, "New Knowledge of Fluorine in Relation to Dental Caries," *J.A.W.W.A.* 31:1926-1930, November 1939. **32.** W. J. Pelton and J. M. Wisan, *Dentistry in Public Health,* Philadelphia, W. B. Saunders Co., 1949. Chapter 8, H. T. Dean, pp. 136-162. **33.** *Hearings Before the House Select Committee,* p. 1647. **34.** *Ibid.,* p. 1642. **35.** *Ibid.,* p. 1637. **36.** H. T. Dean and E. Elvove, "Some Epidemiological Aspects of Chronic Endemic Dental Fluorosis," *Am. J. Pub. Health* 26:567-575, June 1936. **37.** H. T. Dean, "Domestic Water and Dental Caries," *J.A. W.W.A.* 35:1161-1183, September 1943, p. 1176. **38.** C. F. Deatherage, "Mottled Enamel from Standpoint of Public Health

Dentist (including The Relation of Fluorine to Dental Caries in Illinois)," *Fluorine and Dental Health*, A.A.A.S., Washington, D. C., 1942. **39.** N. A. Lange, *Handbook of Chemistry*, Sandusky, Ohio, Handbook Publishers, Inc. 1946, 6th ed., p. 750. **40.** F. A. Arnold, "Fluoride in Drinking Water: Its Effect on Dental Caries," *J.A.D.A.* 36:28-36, January 1948. **41.** H. T. Dean, P. Jay, F. A. Arnold, Jr., and E. Elvove, "Domestic Water and Dental Caries," *Pub. Health Rep.* 56:761-792, April 11, 1941. **42.** H. T. Dean, F. A. Arnold, Jr., and E. Elvove, "Domestic Water and Dental Caries," *Pub. Health Rep.* 57:1155-1179, August 7, 1942. **43.** *Hearings Before the House Select Committee*, p. 1653. **44.** *Ibid.*, pp. 1648, 1649, 1652. **45.** H. T. Dean, "Epidemiological Studies in the United States," *Symposium on Dental Caries and Fluorine*, A.A.A.S., Washington, D. C., 1946, pp. 5-35. Also S. M. Gordon, *Dental Science and Dental Art*, Philadelphia, Lea & Febiger, 1938, Chapter 12. **46.** F. B. Exner, *Hearings Before the Committee on Interstate and Foreign Commerce*, House of Representatives, 83rd Congress, Washington, D. C., Government Printing Office, 1954. **47.** J. G. Frisch, *op. cit.* **48.** Boissevain, *op. cit.* **49.** Schour and Smith, "Experimental Dental Fluorosis." **50.** M. Massler, I. Schour and H. G. Poncher, "Developmental Pattern of the Child as Reflected in the Calcification Pattern of the Teeth," *Am. J. Dis. Child.* 62:3-67, July 1941. **51.** Dean, Jay, Arnold, Elvove, "Domestic Water and Dental Caries." **52.** Deatherage, *op. cit.* **53.** F. J. McClure, "Fluoride Domestic Waters and Systemic Effects," *Pub. Health Rep.* 59:1575-1590, December 8, 1944, p. 1580. **54.** *Hearings Before the Select House Committee*, pp. 1652, 1653. **55.** Dean and Elvove, "Some Epidemiological Aspects of Chronic Endemic Dental Fluorosis." **56.** H. T. Dean, "Investigation of Physiological Effects by Epidemiological Methods," *Fluorine and Dental Health*, A.A.A.S., Washington, D. C., 1942. **57.** *Hearings Before the Committee on Interstate and Foreign Commerce.* **58.** R. G. Agnew and M. C. Agnew, "Environment and Diet, as They Affect Periodontal Structures," *J.A.D.A.* 30:69-80, January 1943. **59.** R. Weaver, "Fluorosis and Dental Caries in Tyneside," *Brit. Dent. J.* 76:29-40, January 21, 1944. **60.** T. Ockerse, "Dental Caries," *Clinical and Experimental Investigation*, Pretoria, Union of South Africa, Government Printer, 1949. **61.** *Ibid.* **62.** Pelton, Wisan, *op. cit.* **63.** H. T. Dean, "Endemic Fluorosis and Its Relation to Dental Caries," *Pub. Health Rep.* 53:1443-1452, August 19, 1938. **64.** H. T. Dean, P. Jay, F. A. Arnold, Jr., F. J. McClure and E. Elvove, "Domestic Water and Dental Caries Including Certain Epidemiological Aspects of Oral L. Acidophilus," *Pub. Health Rep.* 54:862-888, May 26, 1939.

CHAPTER 4

1. F. B. Exner, "Fluoridation," *Northwest Med.* 54:721-737, July 1955. 2. F. B. Exner, "Fluoridation, Part 2," *Northwest Med.* 54:1105-1120, October 1955. 3. Kaj Roholm, *Fluorine Intoxication: A Clinical-hygienic Study*, London, Lewis, 1937. 4. Kaj Roholm, "Fog Disaster in the Meuse Valley, 1930: A Fluorine Intoxication," *J. Ind. Hyg. & Toxicol.* 19:126-136, March 1937. 5. G. J. Cox, "New Knowledge of Fluorine in Relation to Dental Caries," *J.A.W.W.A.* 31:1926-1930, November 1939. 6. M. C. Smith, E. M. Lantz and H. V. Smith, "The Cause of Mottled Enamel," *Science* 74:244, September 4, 1931. 7. H. Velu, "Dystrophie Dentaire des Mammifères des Zones Phosphatées (Darmous) et Fluorose Chronique," *Comp. Rend. Soc. Biol.* 108:750-752, November 21, 1931. 8. H. V. Churchill, "The Occurrence of Fluorides in Some Waters of the United States," *J.A.W.W.A.* 23:1399-1403, September 1931, p. 1399. 9. H. V. Churchill, Discussion of paper by McKay, "Mottled Enamel: A Preventable Endemic Lesion of the Teeth that Presents a New Problem in Civic Responsibility," *J. Dent. Res.* 13:139-143, April 1933. 10. H. V. Churchill, "The Occurrence of Fluorides in Some Waters of the United States." 11. H. T. Dean and F. A. Arnold, Jr., "Endemic Dental Fluorosis or Mottled Enamel," *J.A.D.A.* 35:1278-1283, August 1, 1943. 12. W. J. Pelton and J. M. Wisan, *Dentistry in Public Health*, Philadelphia, W. B. Saunders, 1949. Chapter 8, H. T. Dean, "Fluorine: Water-borne Fluorides and Dental Health." 13. H. T. Dean, "The Investigation of Physiological Effects by the Epidemiological Method," Fluorine and Dental Health, 23-31, A.A.A.S., Washington, D. C., 1942. 14. H. T. Dean, "Chronic Endemic Dental Fluorosis," *J.A.M.A.* 107:1269-1273, October 17, 1936, pp. 1270, 1272. 15. H. T. Dean and E. Elvove, "Studies on the Minimal Threshold of the Dental Sign of Chronic Endemic Fluorosis," *Pub. Health Rep.* 50:1719-1729, December 6, 1935, p. 1719. 16. H. T. Dean, R. M. Dixon and C. Cohen, "Mottled Enamel in Texas," *Pub. Health Rep.* 50:424-442, March 29, 1935. 17. F. B. Exner, Testimony in *Hearings Before the Committee on Interstate and Foreign Commerce*, 83rd Congress, on H. R. 2341: A Bill to Protect the Public Health from the Dangers of Fluorination of Water. 18. H. T. Dean, F. S. McKay and E. Elvove, "Mottled Enamel Survey of Bauxite Arkansas Ten Years After Change in the Common Water Supply," *Pub. Health Rep.* 53:1736-1748, September 30, 1938. 19. H. T. Dean, "Investigation of Physiological Effects by the Epidemiological Method." Also *Hearings Before the House Select Committee to Investigate the Use of Chemicals in Foods and Cosmetics*, House of Representatives, 82nd Congress, Part 3, Washington, D. C., Government Printing

Office, 1952. **20.** N. A. Lange, *Handbook of Chemistry*, Sandusky, Ohio, Handbook Publishers, 6th ed., 1946. **21.** *Hearings Before the House Select Committee*, p. 1507. **22.** *Proceedings, Fourth Annual Conference of State Dental Directors with the Public Health Service and the Children's Bureau*, Federal Security Building, Washington, D. C., June 6-8, 1951. **23.** D. J. Galagan and G. G. Lamson, "Climate and Endemic Dental Fluorosis," *Pub. Health Rep.* 68:497-508, May 1953. **24.** T. P. Parran, "Pioneering for Health: Grand Rapids' Decade of Progress in Fluoridation As An Example," *J.A.D.A.* 51:332-337, September 1955. **25.** *Hearings Before the House Select Committee*, p. 1497. **26.** H. T. Dean, "Epidemiological Studies in the United States," *Dental Caries and Fluorine*, pp. 5-31, Washington, D. C., A.A.A.S., 1946. **27.** *Hearings Before the House Select Committee*. **28.** F. B. Exner, "Physician-patient Relationship," *Northwest Med.* 54:149-155, February 1955. **29.** Editorial, "From Yellow Fever to International Health," *Pub. Health Rep.* 67:1-7, January 1952. **30.** Minutes of a Joint Meeting of Mental Health Committee of Wash. State Med. Assn. and Representatives of County Societies with Representatives of State and Local Health Departments, July 23, 1955. **31.** J. W. Mountin, Editorial, "An Opportunity for Leadership," *Pub. Health Rep.* 66:129-131, February 2, 1951. **32.** F. J. Maier, "Fluoridation of Public Water Supplies," *J.A.W.W.A.* 42:1120-1132, December 1950, p. 1120. **33.** Kaul *vs.* City of Chehalis, 45 Wn. (2d) 616, 635, 277 P. (2d) 352, 362. **34.** Kaul *vs.* City of Chehalis, 45 Wn. (2d) 616, 631, 277 P. (2d) 352, 360. **35.** Kaul *vs.* City of Chehalis, 45 Wn. (2d) 616, 640, 277 P. (2d) 352, 365. **36.** F. B. Exner, *Answer to Open Letter from Roberts Davies, M.D., Medical Director*, Firland San., Seattle, privately published. **37.** G. F. Lull, Editorial, "Fluoridation of Water Supplies," *Today's Health* 33:13, June 1955. **38.** James Madison in a letter to Thomas Jefferson, New York, October 17, 1788. *American State Papers on Freedom of Religion*, Washington, D. C. Religious Liberty Assn., 3rd ed., 1943, p. 181. **39.** Loan Association *vs.* Topeka, 20 Wallace's Reports 655. **40.** *Proceedings of the Atlantic City Meeting*, "Report of the Committee on Hygiene, Public Health and Industrial Health; Res. No. 69," *J.A.M.A.* 158:936, July 16, 1955. **41.** *Hearings Before the Committee on Interstate and Foreign Commerce*, House of Representatives, 83rd Congress, 2nd Session, on H. R. 2341, pp. 277-281. **42.** Dean and Arnold, "Endemic Dental Fluorosis or Mottled Enamel." **43.** Dean, "Investigation of Physiological Effects by the Epidemiological Method." **44.** Dean, "Epidemiological Studies in the United States." **45.** *Hearings Before the Committee on Interstate and Foreign Commerce*, p. 379. **46.** *Ibid.*, p. 402. **47.** Wickard *vs.* Filburn, 317 U. S. 111, 131. **48.** L. A. Scheele, "Report on Programs and Problems, 51st Annual Conference of the Surgeon General of

The Public Health Serv. and the Chief of the Children's Bureau with the State and Territorial Health Officers," *Pub. Health Rep.* 68:174-181, February 1953. **49.** *Ibid.,* p. 177. **50.** *Hearings Before the Committee on Interstate and Foreign Commerce,* p. 399. **51.** *Proceedings, Fourth Annual Conference of State Dental Directors,* p. 32. **52.** J. H. Shaw, *Fluoridation as a Public Health Measure,* A.A.A.S., Washington, D. C., 1954, pp. 36-48. See chapter by G. J. Cox, "Acute Fluoride Poisoning and Crippling Chronic Fluorosis." **53.** Shaw, *op. cit.* See chapter by R. F. Soggnaes, "Relative Merits of Various Fluoridation Vehicles," p. 185. **54.** R. F. Soggnaes, "A Condition Suggestive of Threshold Dental Fluorosis observed in Tristan da Cunha; Part I. Clinical Condition of the Teeth," *J. Dent. Res.* 20:303-313, August 1941, pp. 305-306. **55.** H. C. Hodge, "The Concentration of Fluorides in Drinking Water to Give the Point of Minimum Caries with Maximum Safety," *J.A.D.A.* 40:436-439, April 1950. **56.** J. H. Shaw, *Fluoridation as a Public Health Measure,* Washington, D. C., A.A.A.S., 1954, pp. 79-109. See chapter by H. C. Hodge and F. A. Smith, "Some Public Health Aspects of Fluoridation," pp. 93, 103. **57.** E. R. Schlesinger, "The Safety of Water Fluoridation," *New York Med.* 54:2449-2452, September 1, 1954. **58.** W. Bartlett, H. A. Bulger and R. O. Muether, "Water Fluoridation: Report of the Committee of the St. Louis Medical Society," *Missouri Med.* 51:124-142, February 1954, pp. 128, 130, 135, 136. **59.** F. A. Bull, "Public Health Aspects of Water Fluoridation in Wisconsin," *Fluoridation of Public Water Supplies, A Symposium,* University of Washington, April 27, 1951, pp. 7, 8. **60.** *Hearings Before the Committee on Interstate and Foreign Commerce,* p. 398. **61.** *Proceedings, Fourth Annual Conference of State Dental Directors,* pp. 36-37. **62.** M. E. Nicholson, "The Practicing Dentist's Viewpoint," *J.A.D.A.* 55:144-147, February 1952, p. 147. **63.** M. L. Tainter, "The Promotion of Research," *J.A.D.A.* 30:1239-1240, August 1943. **64.** Statement from California State Department of Health, editorial: "A Second Note on Fluoridation," *Sunnyvale Standard,* October 1, 1954. **65.** Letter to Mrs. Norma Cort, Signed by John E. Zur, Deputy Director, Dept. of Public Health, Illinois, September 13, 1954. **66.** Henry Leicester, Transcription of tape-recording of panel discussion at Jordan Jr. High School, Palo Alto, Calif., October 13, 1954. **67.** Henry Leicester, Transcription of talk at McKinley School, Burlingame, Calif., Feb. 24, 1955. **68.** *Ibid.* **69.** R. V. Lee, C. H. Ellertson, *et al., Give Our Children Better Teeth,* Palo Alto Dental Health Council, Palo Alto, Calif., 1954. **70.** A. P. Black, transcribed testimony before the Florida State Board of Health, Jacksonville, August 20, 1955, pp. 53, 54, 59. **71.** Benjamin Nesin, letter to the Editor, *J.A.D.A.,* June 9, 1955. **72.** Testimony presented to Florida State Board of Health in the presence of Dr. Black, and undisputed.

PART 2

1. The following articles by Dr. G. L. Waldbott on incipient fluoride poisoning are now either in press or ready for publication:

Waldbott, G. L., "Incipient Chronic Fluoride Intoxication from Drinking Water. I. Report on 52 Cases," *Acta Medica Scand.* In press.

Waldbott, G. L., "Incipient Chronic Fluoride Intoxication from Drinking Water. II. Distinction Between Allergic Reactions and Drug Intolerance," *Intern. Arch. of Allergy and Appl. Immun.* In press.

Waldbott, G. L., "Incipient Chronic Fluoride Intoxication from Drinking Water. III. Reproduction of Symptoms during Excretion Studies." Ready for publication.

Waldbott, G. L., "Incipient Chronic Fluoride Intoxication from Drinking Water. IV. Urinary Fluoride and Calcium Excretion in Susceptible Persons." Ready for publication.

Waldbott, G. L., "Tetaniform Convulsions Due to Fluoridated Drinking Water." Ready for publication.

Waldbott, G. L., Dermatological Lesions in Chronic Intoxication from Fluoridated Drinking Water," Munich, *Hautartz.* In press.

CHAPTER 5

1. L. Slagsvold, "Fluoroforgiftning," *Norsk. Vet. Tidsskr.* 46:2, 1934. 2. C. Bartolucci, quoted by K. Roholm in *Fluorine Intoxication,* London, H. K. Lewis & Co., Ltd., 1937. 3. Bulletin #381, National Research Council, *Fluorosis Problem in Livestock Production,* September 1955. 4. K. Roholm, *Fluorine Intoxication,* London, Lewis, 1937. 5. G. L. Waldbott, review, "Medical Evidence Against Fluoridation of Public Water Supplies," *Aust. J. of Dent.* 2:13-20, 1955. 6. S. V. Rao, letter to the editor, *J.A.M.A.* 159:1475, December 10, 1955. 7. O. Lyth, "Endemic Fluorosis in Kweichow, China," the *Lancet* 1:233-235, 1946. 8. John R. Herman, "Fluorine in Urinary Tract Calculi," *Proc. Soc. Exp. Biol. and Med.* 91:189-191, 1956. 9. L. Spira, "Urinary Calculi and Fluorine," *Exp. Med. & Surg.* 14: 73-88, March 1956. 10. G. Frada and G. Mentesana, "Some Observations on Chronic Fluorosis," *Boll. d. I. Soc. Ital. Biol. Sper.* 29:750-53, April 1953. 11. D. C. Leake and G. Ritchie, "Preliminary Note on Blood Picture in Dogs Following Atrophic Gastritis Induced by Sodium Fluoride," *Am. J. Physiol.* 76:234, 1926. 12. E. J. Largent, W. Machle, I. F. Ferneau, "Fluoride Ingestion and Bone Changes in Experimental Animals," *J. Ind. Hyg. and Tox.* 25:396-408, 1943. 13. A. H. Siddiqui, "Fluorosis in Nalgonda District, Hyderabad-Deican," *Brit. Med. J.,* December 10, 1955, pp. 1408-1413. 14. L. Spira, "Etiology of Otosclerosis," *J. of Laryng. and Otol.* 58: 151-157, 1943.

15. J. F. Linsman, C. A. McMurray, "Fluoride Osteosclerosis from Drinking Water," *Radiology* 40:474-84 (misprint corrected in 41:497, 1943). **16.** H. A. Mascheroni, J. M. Munoz, and C. Reussi, "Bone Manifestations of Endemic Fluorosis," *Rev. Soc. Argent. de Biol.* 15:417-19, 1939. **17.** G. L. Waldbott, "Chronic Fluorine Intoxication from Drinking Water at the One Part per Million Concentration. A Case Report," *Int. Arch. of Allergy and Applied Immunology* 7:70-74, 1955. **18.** G. L. Waldbott, "Chronic Fluorine Intoxication from Drinking Water at the One Part per Million Concentration. An Epidemic in Saginaw, Michigan," *Folia Clinica Internacional* 5:144-150, 1955. **19.** Siddiqui, *op. cit.* **20.** Frada and Mentesana, *op. cit.* **21.** Siddiqui, *op. cit.* **22.** S. Murthi, D. Rao, P. Venkateswarly, "Studies of Endemic Fluorosis Compression of the Spinal Cord Due to Skeletal Fluorosis," *Dia. Med.* 27:857-860, May 1955. **23.** R. C. Likins, F. J. McClure and A. C. Steer, "Urinary Excretion of Fluoride Following Defluoridation of a Water Supply," *Pub. Health Rep.* 71:217-22, March 1956. **24.** G. C. Brun, H. Buchwald, and K. Roholm, "Fluorine Excretion in Urine in Chronic Fluorine Poisoning in Cryolite Workers," *Acta Med. Scand.* 106:261-273, 1941. **25.** Siddiqui, *op. cit.* **26.** F. DeEds, "Insecticides, Pest Control Agents and Spray Residues in Relation to the Public Health, Fluorine Toxicity," *Proc. Sixth Pac. Cong. Science* V1, 177-183, 1939. **27.** F. De-Senarclens, "Contribution to the Study of Fluorine Osteoporosis, *Helvetica Med. Acta* 8:379-426, 1941. **28.** DeEds, *op. cit.* **29.** E. L. Largent, "Rates of Elimination of Fluoride Stored in the Tissues of Man," *A.M.A. Arch. Ind. Hyg.* 6:37-42, July 1952. **30.** D. A. Weddle, J. C. Muhler, "The Effect of Inorganic Salts on Fluorine Storage in the Rat, *J. of Nutrition* 34:437-444, 1954. **31.** M. Lawrenz and H. H. Mitchell, "The Relative Assimilation of Fluorine from Fluorine-bearing Minerals and Food (Tea) and from Water and Food," *J. of Nutrition* 22:621, 1941. **32.** J. C. Muhler and H. G. Day, "Effect of pH and State of Oxidation of Different Fluorides in the Drinking Water on Dental Caries and Fluorine Storage in the Rat," *J. of Dent. Res.* 34:68-72, February 1955. **33.** Bulletin #381, National Research Council," *op. cit.* **34.** J. Wilkie, "Two Cases of Fluoride Osteosclerosis," *Br. J. of Radiol.* 13:213-317, 1940. **35.** C. G. Pandit *et al.*, "Spondylosis Deformans in Relation to Fluorine and General Nutrition," the *Lancet* 2:93-96, 1942.

CHAPTER 6

1. Statement by Dr. C. B. Thomas, D.D.S., in Lebanon (Mo.) *Daily Record*, May 3, 1956. **2.** Report of the Dental Committee to the Detroit Commissioner of Health, Dr. J. G. Molner, and submitted to the Detroit Common Council on February 10, 1950. **3.** Letter by Dr.

C. L. Farrell, Pawtucket, R. I., to Dr. G. L. Waldbott, dated October 16, 1954. **4.** Tampa *Sunday Tribune,* December 16, 1951. **5.** "The Problem of Providing Optimum Intake for Prevention of Dental Caries," National Research Council Bulletin #294, November 1953. **6.** E. R. Schlesinger, D. E. Overton, and H. C. Chase, "A Study of Children Drinking Fluoridated and Non-fluoridated Water," *J.A.M.A.* 160:21-24, January 1956. **7.** A. M. Bond and M. M. Murray, "Kidney Structure and Function in Chronic Fluorosis," *Brit. J. Exp. Path.* 33:168, April 1952. **8.** "Report of the Committee of the St. Louis Medical Society," *Missouri Med.,* 1954, pp. 124-142. **9.** C. L. Steinberg *et al., Ann. of Rheum. Dis.* 14:379, 1955. **10.** J. C. Geiger, *California and Western Medicine,* February 1936. **11.** H. Borei, *Inhibition of Cellular Oxidation by Fluoride,* London, Lewis, 1945. **12.** Letter by Dr. H. Borei addressed to Dr. G. L. Waldbott. **13.** Dr. F. DeEds's letter to Dr. G. L. Waldbott dated July 28, 1954. **14.** This was finally published by F. L. Losse in the *Transactions of the American Academy of Nutrition,* 1952. **15.** This is vividly described in a most amazing story by W. R. Cox, *Hello, Test Animals,* Milwaukee, Olsen Pub. Co., 1953. **16.** "Report of the Ad Hoc Committee on Fluoridation," National Research Council Bulletin #214. **17.** Photostats of some of these contracts are in my possession.

CHAPTER 8

1. C. J. Cox, H. L. Dodds, S. F. Dixon and H. C. Matuschak, *J. of Dent. Res.* 18:469, 1939. **2.** F. A. Arnold, *Dental Caries & Fluorine,* A.A.A.S., 1946, pp. 100 and 106. **3.** V. H. Dietz, *J. Dent. for Children,* 4th quarter, 1954, pp. 258-261. **4.** R. Feltman, Personal Communication, July 6, 1956.

INDEX

Index

Abernethy, Thomas G., 220
Agnew, M. C., 112
Agnew, R. G., 112
Akron, Ohio, abandons program, 10
Albany, Oregon, 219
Allergy, to fluorides, 164-167
Aluminum Company of America, 10,
    121, 121 *fn.*, 194
Aluminum utensils, fluoride in, 120
Amarillo, Texas, 62, 68
American Association for the Ad-
    vancement of Science, 50, 51,
    57, 82, 87, 101, 121, 138, 176,
    180, 235
American Association of Dental
    Editors, 138
American Cancer Society, 72
American Dental Association, 4, 6,
    7, 8 *fn.*, 9, 14, 15, 16, 26, 47,
    82, 138, 151, 175, 217, 235,
    246, 247
    propaganda tactics, 188-191
    public relations experts, 189
American Medical Association, 8,
    57, 79, 123, 133, 138, 176, 217
    fluoridation program endorsed,
    136-137, 149-150, 178, 179, 235
    Salk vaccine and the, 136
American Public Health Association,
    8, 8 *fn.*, 93, 94, 100, 138, 176,
    235
American Water Works Associa-
    tion, 8 *fn.*, 101, 138, 151, 179,
    197, 203 *fn.*

America's Health (Ewing), 174
Armstrong, 54, 72, 143, 185
Arnold, F. A., Jr., 103, 176 *fn.*, 211-
    212
Arteriosclerosis, 147
Arthritis, 170
Atlanta, Georgia, 102
Atomic Energy Commission, 55
Aurora, Illinois, 103, 106-108, 110
Authoritarianism, in U. S. Public
    Health Service, 118-153

Baltimore, Maryland, 102
Barden, C. A., 176 *fn.*
Bartlett, Texas, 66, 73-75, 76, 77,
    90-91, 182
Bartolucci, 61
Baton Rouge, Louisiana, abandons
    program, 10
Baumann, A. C., 190
Baumgartner, Leona, 183, 213, 234,
    239
Bauxite, Arkansas, fluoridation pro-
    gram, 45
Beech-Nut Packing Corporation, 21
Bernardi, 78
Biochemical Institute (University of
    Texas), 71
Birmingham, Alabama, 194
Bittner, 185
Black, A. P., 151, 152, 179, 197
Black, G. V., 82, 83, 85, 91
Blandin, Ph. Fr., 84
Blayney, J. R., 59, 117, 143, 178